AF441103

Gut health diet for beginners

Charles Thompson

Copyright© 2020by Charles Thompson

All rights reserved. This document is geared towards providing exact and reliable information with regards to the topic and issue covered. The publication is sold with the idea that the publisher is not required to render accounting, officially permitted, or otherwise, qualified services. If advice is necessary, legal or professional, a practiced individual in the profession should be ordered. - From a Declaration of Principles which was accepted and approved equally by a Committee of the American Bar Association and a Committee of Publishers and Associations. In no way is it legal to reproduce, duplicate, or transmit any part of this document in either electronic means or in printed format. Recording of this publication is strictly prohibited and any storage of this document is not allowed unless with written permission from the publisher. All rights reserved. The information provided herein is stated to be truthful and consistent, in that any liability, in terms of inattention or otherwise, by any usage or abuse of any policies, processes, or directions contained within is the solitary and utter responsibility of the recipient reader. Under no circumstances will any legal responsibility or blame be held against the publisher for any reparation, damages, or monetary loss due to the information herein, either directly or indirectly. Respective authors own all copyrights not held by the publisher. The information herein is offered for informational purposes solely, and is universal as so. The presentation of the information is without contract or any type of guarantee assurance.

The trademarks that are used are without any consent, and the publication of the trademark is without permission or backing by the trademark owner. All trademarks and brands within this book are for clarifying purposes only and are the owned by the owners themselves, not affiliated with this document.

Contents

Gut health diet for beginners

Introduction

A healthy gut it essential for our well-being. When it works well, we have an edge, while when something is wrong, we realize it immediately. The intestine is a very important organ. It contains digestion and absorption of food, but it also has an immune function and many metabolic functions. Its balance is very delicate and depends on various factors, mainly attributable to our lifestyle. A diet rich in sugars, fats, alcoholic beverages, and excessive use of drugs is a risk factor that puts a strain on our intestines and stresses; it is now well established that the psychological state plays a decisive role in our state health. When bowel problems tend to recur, it is advisable to run for cover. "Gut Health Diet for Beginners" offers numerous useful information and a tasty recipe book designed for a diet that contrasts intestinal pain without sacrificing the pleasure of the table.

Chapter 1: Gut health

All food is broken down in the intestine into a simple form that can enter the bloodstream and be transported as a nutrient throughout our body. This is only possible with a healthy and functional digestive system. A healthy gut contains good bacteria and immune cells that ward off infectious agents, such as germs, viruses, and fungi. A healthy gut also communicates with the brain through nerves and hormones, which helps maintain mental and physical health and well-being. There is a close link between intestinal health and the emotional sphere, and vice versa: let's think about how much stress can affect, causing manifestations such as spastic colitis, gastritis, digestive difficulties.

The signs that something is wrong

Everyone can suffer from digestive problems like abdominal pain, bloating, loose stools, constipation, heartburn, nausea, or vomiting at some point for a while. When symptoms persist (it's helpful to call your doctor), they could be a sign of an underlying problem that needs medical investigation. Weight loss for no good reason, blood in stools, black stools (a sign of bleeding in the gut), severe vomiting associated with fever, severe stomach pain, difficulty swallowing food, pain in the throat or chest when eating ingested or jaundice (recognizable when the skin and/or eyes turn yellow) could potentially indicate a gastrointestinal problem with more severe consequences that need to be established.

Factors that affect intestinal health

The factors that can soothe the health of our intestines are the inexorable advancing age or during pregnancy. In fact, due to aging - within certain limits - a slowing of intestinal motility and the appearance of a sluggish intestine is to be considered everyday phenomena. The same goes for pregnancy, during which the woman's body undergoes numerous changes, both at the hormonal and physical level, which can favor the decrease of intestinal motility, giving rise to a lazy intestine problem.

However, in individuals not affected by the aforementioned physiological conditions, intestinal health can be compromised:

• Incorrect feeding;

• Insufficient water supply;

• Conditions of psychophysical stress (excessive rhythms of work or study, worries, nervous conditions, etc.);

• Sedentary life;

• Diseases of the enteric tract (eg, irritable bowel syndrome, etc.);

• Taking or misusing certain types of drugs (for example, antihypertensive drugs, antidepressants, antacids, etc.).

When to worry?

As a result of stressful situations or in the presence of an unregulated lifestyle, our intestine condition can be compromised and can be resolved through simple behavioral measures. Notwithstanding the importance of the medical examination, if the disorder is resolved in a short time, by merely paying attention to diet and personal habits, it should not worry. On the contrary, if the intestinal disorders occur suddenly with no apparent cause (no stress, correct nutrition, a good level of physical activity) and/or if it is associated with unusual symptoms - such as fatigue, fever, very intense abdominal pain, presence of blood in the stool, etc. - it is important to contact a doctor immediately to identify the possible presence of pathologies not yet identified. Therefore, in such situations, the lazy bowel could represent the symptom of a disease affecting the enteric tract.

Chapter 2: Diet for a healthy intestine

The goal of the diet for a healthy intestine must be to reactivate normal intestinal motility. It can be useful to increase your fiber intake by consuming vegetables, legumes, cereals, and some types of fruit. Be careful, however, to also ensure an adequate supply of water. Increasing the fiber in your diet without drinking the right amounts of water can lead to a counterproductive result for which the condition of the intestine worsens further. Furthermore, an excessively high-fiber diet could interfere with other nutrients' absorption, causing various problems and disorders. Therefore, yes to the fibers, but without e xaggerating.

Food for the gut

Here is an overview of foods that can help your gut stay healthy. The recommendation is not to focus on these foods and not to forget the respect of seasonality; Furthermore, it is good to underline the natural choice's importance. The absence of pesticides is of great help when you want to move from a pathological to a non-pathological ecosystem.

Oats: It has a high content of soluble fibers, which fight constipation and stimulate peristaltic movements. Oats, an excellent cereal that must never be missing in a healthy intestinal breakfast, can shield the intestinal bacterial flora. It has a low glycemic index and is therefore also suitable for people with diabetes.

Persimmon: fights intestinal inflammation.

Apple: here, the merit is of a soluble fiber that regulates intestinal transit (obviously you have to drink!): It is the pectin contained in apples which, baked in the oven, are allied foods of the intestine.

Raw artichokes: useful in intestinal infections and chronic diarrhea.

Carrot: anti-putrid regulates the intestine and helps the mucosa to heal; the black one contains quality antioxidants which, thanks to the fibers, are absorbed in the colon, where they perform an antitumor action.

Cabbage: healing and anti-inflammatory, excellent in the form of juice even with carrot; two leaves, wrapped in wool, flare up if kept on the stomach for the night.

Blueberry: antiseptic, fights fermentation and dysentery.

Miso: derived from soy, it is rich in enzymes useful for gastrointestinal well-being. Excellent in the form of soup.

Barley: refreshing and emollient, it promotes intestinal transit.

Potato: emollient for the mucous membranes promotes bowel function, fights constipation and hemorrhoids.

Rice: wholemeal is anti-fermentative and anticolitic; it also contains tricine, a substance that counteracts the synthesis of eicosanoids (biological agents linked to inflammatory processes). The polished rice, or rather its cooking water, slows down diarrhea.

Buckwheat (wheat): rich in antioxidants, it is strongly anti-inflammatory.

Flax seeds: rich in fiber and antioxidants, they must be ground at the moment of use with a coffee grinder and added to yogurt, fruit, salads, or others. Try them, for example, with an apple and a little brown rice milk.

Yogurt with Probiotics: at the supermarket refrigerated counter, choose yogurt enriched with live lactic ferments (it must be specified on the label). They are beneficial as they are rich in good bacteria that enhance bacteria's work already naturally present in our intestine.

Extra Virgin Olive Oil: it is the healthiest condiment par excellence, the cornerstone of the Mediterranean diet. Two teaspoons a day, to dress salads or vegetables or, again, to add to pasta sauce preparation, will contribute to intestinal health because this food can convert insoluble fiber into a highly digestible fiber. It is also valuable because it lubricates and nourishes the intestine from within.

Fennel: the detox vegetable that must never be missing on our tables (especially before, during, and after the holidays!). Fennel is a mine of fibers with digestive and antispasmodic properties. Due to their purifying function, they can counteract air formation in the belly, helping the person get rid of bloating, aerophagia, diarrhea, colic, and intestinal cramps.

Foods rich in Omega 3: foods such as flax seeds, walnuts, salmon, sardines, mackerel, avocado are anti-inflammatory foods, thanks to the concentration of beneficial fatty acids for the body. In particular, they act on the intestinal mucosa as a natural emollient, facilitating intestinal transit.

Kiwi: they promote and increase intestinal transit, which is why they are useful in the case of constipation and chronic constipation.

Asparagus: a concentrate of fibers particularly effective in stimulating and regulating intestinal transit.

Water: it is not a food, but it is essential to hydrate and drink at least one and a half / two liters a day. Water cleans and treats the intestine as it allows the elimination of toxins and residues left inside the colon.

Useful tips for having a healthy intestine

The best strategy that can be implemented for a healthy intestine is the preventive one. Except for the presence of any diseases of the enteric tract that cannot always be prevented, following small behavioral precautions can prove to be an excellent stratagem to avoid facing complications of intestinal motility. In light of what has been said so far, therefore, it is possible to state that to prevent the appearance of a lazy intestine, it can be useful:

- Follow a balanced diet, characterized by the right amount of fiber and always accompanied by an adequate water intake.
- Avoid both physical and psychological stress, trying to reduce, as much as possible, the work and study rhythms if excessive, removing the states of anxiety and nervousness.
- Engage in regular physical activity. Movement contributes to the well-being and maintenance of bowel motility. In addition to this, constant physical activity helps to release tensions, relaxing the body and mind.
- Support the evacuation stimulus. Many people, especially when away from home, tend to hold back and ignore the urge to avoid using public toilets. However, this behavior, mostly if continued for long periods, can favor the slowing of intestinal transit and the appearance of a sluggish intestine.
- Adequate sleep is essential for gut health. It is not uncommon for people with sleep disorders to suffer from nausea, bloating, constipation, and other digestive problems.
- Avoid fried foods and consume alcohol and caffeine in moderation, as they are not healthy in the long run. Avoid fried foods, drink alcohol and caffeine in moderation, as they are not beneficial in the long run.

Chapter 3: Breakfast

1) Crêpes of chickpea flour with cabbage and fermented cashew nuts

Ingredients:

For the crêpes:

- 280 g of chickpea flour
- 500 ml of warm water
- 40 g of extra virgin olive oil
- 4 g cumin seeds
- 4 g sage
- 8 g of whole salt
- 10 cabbage leaves.

For the cashew spread:

- 150 g raw cashews
- 20 g white miso
- 8 g lemon juice
- 10 g nutritional yeast
- 3 g of whole salt
- 3 g yellow mustard powder
- water q.s.

For the crêpes: with the help of a whisk, mix the chickpea flour, water, and 20 g of extra virgin olive oil. Leave to rest for at least 8 hours. Then pick up the dough and season it with a mix obtained by blending the cumin, sage, and salt. Mix well. Heat a non-stick or iron pot well, pour a teaspoon of sunflower oil, and distribute it well over the entire surface. Pour a ladle of batter, cook it until it comes off, then turn it over and cook it on the other side as well. When it is ready, place it on absorbent food paper and proceed with the dough. Cut the cabbage leaves thin. Heat a wok-like pan with the remaining extra virgin olive oil. Sauté the cabbage for a few minutes, add salt and let the vegetation water evaporate and it will come out. Keep them aside. For the spread: soak the cashews for 12 hours at room temperature, changing the water at least a couple of times. After that, rinse them well and put them in a blender along with all the ingredients. Blend until the mixture is creamy and without lumps. Serve the crêpes with the cabbage, a few flakes of cashew spread, and grated black pepper.

2) Almond cookies

Ingredients:
- **400 g of peeled almonds**
- **400 g of light brown sugar**
- **100 g of powdered sugar**
- **50 g of flour**
- **2 egg whites**
- **20 g of water**
- **1 teaspoon of yeast**

Finely chop the almonds with 350 g of brown sugar. In a saucepan, over low heat, dissolve 50 g of sugar in 20 g of water. When the syrup is ready, add it to the almond mixture and the yeast, flour, and 50 g of powdered sugar. The mixture obtained must rest at room temperature for at least 12 hours covered with a damp cloth. After 12 hours, whisk the egg whites with 50 g of powdered sugar and mix them with the almond mixture (they are gradually incorporated by mixing them from the bottom up). Work until it is soft and homogeneous. Obtain some loaves that you will cut into small pieces and to which you will give the shape of the almond. Bake in the oven at 110 ° for about ten minutes. Let cool before serving with a sprinkling of icing sugar. Store them in a tin box to keep them longer.

3)   Chocolate, almond, nut and coconut cookies

Ingredients:
- **100 g of dark chocolate**
- **50 g of shelled almonds**
- **50 g of walnut kernels**
- **30 g of shredded coconut**
- **50 g of whole coconut sugar**
- **1 egg white whipped until stiff**
- **the peel of 1 organic orange**
- **1 pinch of salt**

Put the diced chocolate and the other dry ingredients, including the orange peel, in the mixer. Blend everything for a few minutes until it is reduced to a powder. You will get a rather lumpy mixture. Meanwhile, whip the egg white until stiff and add it to the dough, mixing carefully. Using a spoon, form balls of the mixture and place them on a baking tray lined with parchment paper. Try to distance them from each other because they will widen during cooking. Bake the cookies at 150 ° for 25 minutes. Let them cool before removing them.

4)   Stuffed chickpea flour pancakes

Ingredients:
- 3 heaping tablespoons of spelled flour
- 2 heaping tablespoons of corn starch
- 3 heaping tablespoons of chickpea flour
- 2 tablespoons of oil and 1 pinch of salt
- 1 pinch of nutmeg
- 300 ml of partially skimmed milk

For the stuffing
- 1 small thistle (about 200 g) already cleaned
- 1 slice of clean pumpkin
- ½ small leek
- 2 teaspoons of flour
- 2 teaspoons of lemon juice
- 4 tablespoons of oil and 1 pinch of salt

For the batter: dissolve the flour and starch in a little milk, then gradually pour the remaining liquid and oil, beating with a whisk. When the cream is thick and fluid, add the salt and nutmeg. Let it sit for 20-30 minutes.

For the filling: blanch the thistle in 500 ml of water where you have diluted the lemon and flour. Wash the leek and slice it thinly. Sauté it in a pan with 1 tablespoon of oil and 3 of water for 4-5 minutes, then add the coarsely grated pumpkin and the shredded thistle. After another 4-5 minutes turn off the heat.

Mix the batter. Just grease a non-stick pan and pour a ladle of the mixture into a thin layer. Cook the crepes for a few minutes on both sides. Stuff them and close them in a bundle. Serve hot.

5)   Buckwheat pancakes with nettle sauce

Ingredients:
- **250 g of buckwheat flour**
- **150 g of nettle tops**
- **400 ml of soy milk**
- **3 tablespoons of white flour**
- **oil**
- **salt**

Put the flour in a bowl with the water needed to have a semi-fluid batter. Add salt, stir and let it rest for 30 minutes. Wash the nettles and blanch them for 5 minutes in a little salted water. Remove them with a slotted spoon and set them aside. Measure out 100 ml of their liquid (save the rest for other preparations). First, toast the white flour in a saucepan; first, pour the hot nettle water and then, always stirring and, little by little, the previously heated milk. Let the sauce thicken over low heat, then add the coarsely chopped nettles. Season with salt and season with a tablespoon and a half of oil. Heat a little oil in a pan and cook a ladle of batter at a time until you have not too thin crepes. Serve with the nettle sauce.

6)   Savory pie with red lentils

Ingredients:

For the base (pan diameter 24 cm)

- 250 g wholemeal flour
- 3 tablespoons of extra virgin olive oil
- a teaspoon of natural yeast
- a teaspoon of whole sea salt
- water q.s.

For the filling

- 3 medium potatoes
- 2 glasses of red lentils
- a clove of garlic
- a slice of ginger
- half a small pepper
- 2 sage leaves
- extra virgin olive oil as needed
- whole sea salt to taste
- water or vegetable broth to taste

To garnish the surface of the cake

- Sesame seeds
- poppy seeds
- chopped almonds to taste

In a large bowl, pour the flour, salt, and yeast and mix well. Make a hole in the center in which to put the oil and, a little at a time, the water needed to knead. Work vigorously until you have obtained a compact but soft, elastic, and not stiff dough. Let it rest for 30 minutes in the fridge. In a saucepan, boil some water with a handful of coarse salt and the unpeeled potatoes. Cook them until they are soft. Drain them, let them cool and peel them. With a puree or a fork, mash them well. Mix well and set aside. In the meantime, put a drizzle of oil in a saucepan, heat and fry the whole clove of crushed garlic and the chili pepper, add a little water, then add the finely chopped ginger, the sage, and the lentils previously washed under running water. Mix well and add the hot water or vegetable broth necessary to cover the lentils. Salt. Set aside more hot water or broth, which will be added during cooking. Usually, in 15-20 minutes, they are cooked, do not worry if they fall apart slightly. The flavor given to the cake does not vary. After cooking, let them cool. Roll out your base with the help of a rolling pin until you get an elastic dough, not too thin because it must support and give body to the cake. Line a baking sheet with parchment paper and lay the base on top, cutting off the excess edge, which you can use to prepare decorative strips for the surface. After removing the garlic and sage leaves, add the lentils to the potatoes. Mix well, seasoning with salt. Place the filling on the base, pour over a cascade of sesame seeds, chopped almonds, and poppy seeds. If you want, lay the puff pastry strips on top of the cake, forming the characteristic grid. Add a drizzle of oil on the surface and bake at 200 ° for about 40 minutes. Let it cool down a bit before serving. This savory pie is excellent when accompanied by raw and cooked seasonal vegetables.

7) Savory pie with potatoes and creamy mushrooms

Ingredients:
- 250 g of wholemeal flour
- 3 tablespoons of sourdough
- soya milk
- 1 teaspoon of brown sugar
- 2 tablespoons of oil
- 6 medium potatoes
- 200 g of mushrooms
- 100 g of sour cream
- 150 g of ricotta
- 2 cloves of garlic
- 1 teaspoon of marjoram
- 2 teaspoons of sweet paprika
- sea salt

Mix the flour with the sourdough, a little salt, and the lukewarm milk necessary to have a firm and homogeneous dough. Knead it for a long time on a table, wrap it into a ball and let it rise in a warm place for 4-5 hours. Meanwhile, wash the potatoes and steam them with the peel. While these are getting warm, peel the mushrooms and stew them in a pan with minced garlic, paprika, marjoram, and a little salt. When soft, add the cream and crumbled goat cheese. Peel the potatoes and cut them into slices about 1 cm thick. Roll out two thirds of the dough and use it to line a floured, rectangular, or round, high mold. Spread the potatoes inside, cover with mushrooms. Roll out the rest of the dough so that it covers the entire surface. Seal the edges well, brush with a little warm milk and bake at 180 degrees for 30-35 minutes. Serve the cake hot.

8)   Energy cookies with oats and raisins

Ingredients:
- **300 g of rolled oats**
- **100 g of raisins**
- **the grated zest of a lemon**
- **the zest of a grated orange**
- **150 g of rice malt**
- **a teaspoon of ground cinnamon**
- **a teaspoon of vanilla powder**
- **apple juice to taste**

First, soak the raisins in warm water for about 15 minutes, turn on the oven at 180 ° and prepare a pan lined with parchment paper to lay the biscuits to cook them. Once this is done, you can dedicate yourself to the dough, starting with toasting the oat flakes in a hot pan for a few minutes, stirring often. Place them still hot in a large bowl in which you will add the grated citrus peel, cinnamon, vanilla powder, and finally, the well squeezed raisins. At this point, add the malt to the mixture; knead with your hands with the help of a little apple juice (just enough to be able to work the dough without making it too liquid). You can proceed by taking some of the dough to form balls that you will crush in your hands to give it the classic shape of a round biscuit. During this step, you can help yourself by wetting your hands with water. Place each biscuit in the pan and bake for about 10-15 minutes. Remove the pan from the oven and let the cookies cool. When they are cold, you can store them in an airtight jar, where they will keep well for a whole week.

9)   Soft fruit plumcake

Ingredients:
- **300 g of buckwheat flour**
- **80 g of sugar**
- **1 sachet of yeast**
- **5 tablespoons of oil**
- **2 egg whites**
- **the zest of 1 grated lemon**
- **1 jar of low-fat yogurt**
- **100 g of shelled walnuts**
- **fresh berries (blueberries, currants, raspberries)**

Mix the flour, sugar, oil, and yeast in a bowl, stir in the yogurt and lemon zest. Separately, whisk the egg whites and add them gently to the previous ingredients. Finally, mix the walnuts and berries into the mixture. Line a loaf pan with baking paper and pour the mixture. Bake at 180 degrees for about 40 minutes. If you want, you can serve this dessert with more low-fat yogurt and some fresh fruit.

10) Omelette with potatoes and onions

Ingredients:
- **800 g of potatoes**
- **6 eggs**
- **2 onions**
- **2 cloves of garlic**
- **2 tablespoons of oil**
- **1 pinch of nutmeg**
- **1 pinch of parsley**
- **1 pinch of chives**
- **pepper**
- **salt**

Finely slice the onions and garlic. Wash and peel the potatoes and cut them into cubes. Fry the onions and garlic in a pan with olive oil and water, add the potatoes, and cook them until tender. Season with the chopped parsley and chives and mix well. Beat the eggs, add the grated nutmeg to taste, and pour the mixture over the potatoes. When the eggs have hardened, turn the omelette and finish cooking on the other side. Serve immediately.

11) Oat porridge with chocolate, cashew and orange

Ingredients:
- **about 10 tablespoons of oat flakes**
- **a few pinches of ground cinnamon**
- **a few pinches of vanilla powder**
- **2 tablespoons of rice syrup**
- **6-7 cashews**
- **dark chocolate to taste**
- **almond milk**
- **a slice of orange**

Put the oat flakes in a bowl, then pour enough milk to cover them abundantly. Let it rest in the fridge overnight. The next morning add the cinnamon, vanilla, rice syrup and mix well. Add more milk if necessary. Complete with crumbled or chopped cashews, dark chocolate into small pieces, and a slice of orange. Consume the porridge immediately.

12) Plum gluten-free muffins

Ingredients:
- **300 g of cooked prunes**
- **4 eggs**
- **150 g of brown sugar**
- **190 g of potato starch**
- **200 g of rice flour**
- **1 vanilla pod**

Whisk the whole eggs with the sugar and the seeds of the vanilla pod. Add the starch, flour, and plums with their liquid to the mixture. Mix well and arrange everything in lightly oiled cups or silicone muffin molds; you should get 7-10 muffins depending on the molds' size. Bake in the oven at 180-190 ° for about 25 minutes, or until it comes out dry by inserting a toothpick inside the cake.

13) Pear, chocolate and hazelnut muffins

Ingredients:
- 3 cups of kamut
- 2 tablespoons of cream of tartar
- half a teaspoon of ground cinnamon
- half a cup of toasted hazelnuts
- half a cup of dark chocolate
- half a cup of sunflower oil
- half a cup of wheat malt
- 1 and a half cups of soy milk
- 1 large cup of pears in small pieces
- 1 pinch of salt

Mix the flour, salt, cream of tartar, and cinnamon in a bowl; in another, emulsify the oil with the malt and milk, then pour it into the first, mixing everything without stirring much. Add the coarsely chopped hazelnuts and chocolate, the peeled and chopped pears. Spread the mixture into muffin cups and bake at 180 degrees for about 30 minutes.

Note: In this recipe, one cup is approximately 120 grams.

14)

Pancakes without butter

Ingredients:
- **Low-fat white yogurt 125 g**
- **00 flour 150 g**
- **Skimmed milk 200 g**
- **Eggs 1**
- **Powdered yeast for cakes 8 g**
- **Extra virgin olive oil q.s.**

Start by placing the egg in a bowl and beating it with a whisk. When it is light and fluffy, add the milk slowly and, continue to beat, add the yogurt. Then add, passing it through a sieve, the flour, and the baking powder. Proceed by mixing carefully, with gentle movements from the bottom to the top, to not disassemble the mixture, until you get a smooth and homogeneous batter. Cover with cling film, and place it in the fridge to rest for about 30 minutes. After this time, recover the batter and heat a non-stick pan with a drizzle of oil over medium heat. Pour a spoonful of batter into the center of the pan, letting it spread by itself. After a few minutes, when small bubbles begin to bloom on the surface, it is time to turn the pancake with the help of a spatula. So cook it for another minute and when it's ready, place it on a plate. Continue like this until the batter is used up. Serve your butter-free pancakes with honey!

15) Gluten free sponge cake

Ingredients:
- **Eggs 5**
- **Brown sugar 150 g**
- **Vanilla bean 1**
- **Corn starch gluten free 150 g**

Start by placing the eggs in a planetary mixer, then add the sugar and whisk the ingredients for at least 10/15 minutes with a whisk until the mixture is frothy, puffy, and light yellow. If you wish, when the mixture is well whipped, you can add the seeds of the vanilla pod that you have cut in half and continue whipping for a few seconds to mix it well and flavor the mixture. At this point, you can add the starch (or potato starch) that you have previously well sieved: mix everything with a wooden spoon until you get a homogeneous mixture, being careful not to dismantle it. Grease and flour a round pan with a diameter of 24 cm with the starch, pour the dough into the mold's center, leveling it well. Bake the gluten-free sponge cake for about 35-40 minutes at 180 ° C in a preheated static oven without ever opening the oven in the first half-hour of cooking. Remove the mold from the oven and let the sponge cake cool in the mold before opening it.

Chapter 4: Snacks, appetizers and side dishes

1) Brussels sprouts with pears and walnuts

Ingredients
- **350 g of Brussels sprouts**
- **40 g of leek**
- **1 small pear**
- **60 g of shelled walnuts**
- **2 juniper berries**
- **salt**
- **4 tablespoons of oil**

Clean and wash the vegetables. Remove the most damaged leaves from the sprouts and divide them into four wedges; add them to the finely sliced leek, which you will dry for 5 minutes in a pan with 2 tablespoons of oil, half a glass of water, and the juniper. Cut the pear into cubes and coarsely chop the walnuts; add them to the mixture and continue cooking for another 3 minutes. Before removing from the heat, season with salt, season with the remaining oil, and stir.

2) Slices of crispy bread with black cabbage and beans

Ingredients:
- **200 grams of dry beans**
- **300 grams of black cabbage**
- **10 slices of wholemeal bread**
- **7-8 cm of kombu seaweed**
- **a few sage leaves**
- **3 cloves of garlic**
- **extra virgin olive oil as needed**
- **Salt and Pepper To Taste**

Soak the beans overnight, remove the soaking water and cook them in plenty of cold water, with the kombu, sage and a clove of garlic, possibly in an earthenware pot, for about two hours or until tender. Low fire. Season with salt and pepper in the last 10 minutes of cooking; remove the kombu, sprinkle the beans with a drizzle of oil and set aside. Meanwhile, peel the black cabbage by removing the fibrous central rib, wash it well and cook the leaves immersed in lightly salted water, until tender (the black cabbage can be more or less tough). Drain, season with oil and a grind of pepper. Place the slices of bread in the oven and brown them on both sides. Rub them immediately with the remaining garlic. Place them on a serving dish and cover with the beans and black cabbage. Serve immediately.

3) Broccoli with miso sauce and nuts

Ingredients:
- **2-3 broccoli tops**
- **80 g of walnuts**
- **2 tablespoons of miso**
- **about 1 cm of ginger root**

Cut and wash the broccoli tops and place them in the steamer basket, adding a pinch of salt. Cook in a covered pot until the broccoli is tender but still bright green. Meanwhile, toast the walnuts in the oven at 180 ° until they are fragrant. Let them cool down. Chop them coarsely by hand to prevent them from releasing too much oil, and then grind them in a mixer with miso and water or vegetable broth, just enough to obtain a smooth cream. Flavor with the ginger juice, obtained by squeezing the grated root. Serve the vegetables with the sauce.

4) Tofu with pear and spinach

Ingredients:
- **200 g of natural tofu**
- **2-3 large handfuls of fresh spinach**
- **1 ripe but firm pear**
- **½ leek**
- **3-4 tablespoons of oil**
- **2-3 tablespoons of tamari**
- **lemon juice, to taste**
- **whole sea salt, to taste**

Clean the vegetables and slice the leek into more or less thin slices. Wash the pear and cut it into pieces. In a heavy-bottomed pan, heat the oil over high heat, add the tamari, and let the leek dry. Also, add the tofu cut into cubes and let it brown on all sides, turning often. Remove from the heat and transfer the tofu with leeks to a salad bowl along with the cleaned spinach and pear slices. Season with the oil of olive to taste, lemon juice and salt, mix and serve.

5) Sweet and sour stewed pumpkin

Ingredients:
- 3 cups of chopped pumpkin
- 2 tablespoons of extra virgin olive oil
- chopped sage to taste
- water q.s.
- 2 tablespoons of rice vinegar
- salt

Heat the oil in a pot with the chopped sage and rosemary, then add the pumpkin, a little salt and sauté for a few minutes. Add a little water and vinegar, cover, and let it simmer over low heat for about 15-20 minutes until the pumpkin is tender.

6) Sweet potato with coriander and curry with ginger and citrus sauce

Ingredients:
- 900 g of sweet potatoes
- 300 ml of vegetable cream
- lemon juice
- the grated zest of 1 lemon
- 6 cm of fresh ginger root
- 4-5 tablespoons of oil
- half a tablespoon of coriander powder
- half a tablespoon of curry powder
- sea salt to taste
- fresh parsley, to taste
- freshly ground black pepper, to taste

Preheat the oven to 180 degrees. Wash the potatoes well, but don't peel them. Cut them into wedges lengthwise and arrange them on a baking tray that you have lined with baking paper. Brush the potatoes

with oil, season with coriander, curry, pepper, salt, and bake.
Meanwhile, prepare the sauce by mixing the vegetable cream, lime
juice, lemon zest, peeled and grated ginger, and salt in a bowl. Set the
sauce aside. Remove the potatoes from the oven when they are tender
and golden and serve with a little sauce and the freshly chopped
parsley.

7) Quick pizzas

Ingredients:
For the dough
- **200 g of finely ground millet**
- **200 g of rice flour**
- **3 tablespoons of oil**
- **1 teaspoon of salt**
- **1 tablespoon yeast**
- **1 tablespoon of sesame and flax seeds**

For the filling:
- **500 g of clean pumpkin**
- **1 sprig of sage**
- **1 sprig of rosemary**
- **2 tablespoons of oil**

For the mini pizzas: Finely chop the seeds. Combine them with the other
ingredients in a large bowl and knead with your hands to get a soft and
homogeneous mixture. Let it rest for about 1 hour. For the filling. Cut
the pumpkin into cubes, sprinkle with chopped sage and rosemary.
Cook it in steam or the oven for 15-20 minutes, let it cool, and season
with oil. Blend it until you have a cream, helping you if needed with a
little water. Roll out the not too thin dough with a rolling pin and cut out
discs with the help of a glass; place them on a baking sheet lined with
parchment paper and cover with the cream. Bake at 170 degrees for
about 15 minutes.

8)   Mushrooms with orange spinach

Ingredients:
- **400 g of fresh spinach leaves**
- **150 g of champignon mushrooms**
- **2 large handfuls of shelled almonds**
- **the juice of 1 blond orange**
- **oil**
- **white pepper, to taste**
- **pink Himalayan salt, to taste**

Clean the spinach and the mushrooms, which you will then have to slice thinly. Put the vegetables in a bowl with the peeled and chopped almonds and mix well. Season with orange juice, oil, a few pinches of Himalayan salt, and freshly ground pepper. Stir again and serve.

9)   Quinoa with roasted carrots

Ingredients:

- **250 g of quinoa**

- **4-5 carrots**

- **4 shallots**

- **1/2 tablespoon of cumin**

- **1/2 tablespoon of turmeric**

- **1 handful of toasted pine nuts**

- **1 handful of parsley and very finely chopped celery**

- **extra virgin olive oil**

- **salt and pepper**

Peel the shallots and halve them; cut the carrots in four lengthwise and then into chunks. Put the vegetables in a pan seasoned with oil, cumin, and salt. Bake at 180 degrees for about 30 minutes, turning them now and then until they are well roasted. Meanwhile, wash the quinoa well in cold water, drain it in a tightly meshed colander and rinse again; drain well and dry briefly in a pan with two tablespoons of oil, turmeric, and pepper. Pour in boiling water equal to double the quinoa's volume, add salt, cover, and cook over very low heat for 15-20 minutes until the liquid is completely absorbed. Shell the quinoa well and mix it with the vegetables, also collecting their cooking juices, with the pine nuts, celery, and parsley. Serve immediately.

10) Spinach in a pan with dried fruit

Ingredients:

- **500 g of spinach**
- **50 g of dried apples**
- **50 g of raisins**
- **a little pine nuts**
- **1 clove of garlic**
- **extra virgin olive oil as needed**
- **Salt to taste**

Soak the apples and raisins for about 20 minutes in warm water. Clean and wash the spinach. Blanch them in lightly salted water for a few minutes. Drain them by squeezing them well, and cut them coarsely. Fry the garlic in a pan greased with oil, add the spinach, and after a while, the raisins and well-squeezed apples, pine nuts, and salt. Let it cook over high heat for a few minutes, season with salt, and serve the spinach hot.

11) Rice and zucchini croquettes with saffron sauce

Ingredients:

For the croquettes:

- **350 g of rice**
- **850 ml of water**
- **800 g of zucchini**
- **2 tablespoons of oil**
- **1 teaspoon of salt**
- **1 bunch of parsley**
- **1 clove of garlic**
- **salt and pepper**

For the saffron sauce:

- **250 ml of soy milk**
- **30 ml of oil**
- **30 g of rice flour**
- **1 sachet of saffron**

Brown the chopped garlic and parsley in a little oil. Add and stew the sliced zucchini with salt and pepper for 10 minutes. Puree about 1/3 of the zucchini. Wash the rice, drain it and cook it in salted water, covered and without stirring, for about 35 minutes. Season the rice with the salt, the zucchini not pureed, stir, and continue cooking for another 5 minutes. Let it cool, then form some meatballs that you will bake in the oven at 200 ° for about 15-20 minutes. To prepare the sauce, brown the flour in a saucepan with the oil, then add the milk. Bring to a boil and let it thicken over low heat, stirring with a whisk. Salt and add the saffron and the zucchini puree.

12) Sweet and sour peppers

Ingredients:

- **2 yellow peppers**
- **2 red peppers**
- **80 g of raisins**
- **100 ml of apple cider vinegar**
- **5 tablespoons of oil**
- **4 cardamom capsules**
- **1-2 tablespoons of chopped parsley**
- **1 teaspoon of turmeric**
- **1 pinch of Himalayan salt**

In a pan with a diameter of 24 cm, heat 200 ml of water with the washed but not soaked raisins, apple cider vinegar, and 2 tablespoons of oil. Meanwhile, clean the peppers well, removing the seeds and white filaments, wash them, and cut them into eight wedges.

Dip them into the boiling liquid along with the cardamom. Cook them for 10 minutes, turn off the stove, season with salt, turmeric, and the remaining oil. Stir and serve sprinkled with chopped parsley.

13) Buckwheat medallions in tomato sauce

Ingredients:

- **200 g of buckwheat**

- **1 clove of squeezed garlic**

- **salt**

- **½ tablespoon of curry**

- **½ tablespoon of marjoram**

- **½ tablespoon of cumin**

- **breadcrumbs**

- **extra virgin olive oil for frying**

For the sauce

- **1 small onion**

- **400 g of tomato puree**

- **1 bunch of basil**

- **salt and pepper**

- **10 pitted olives**

- **2 tablespoons of oil**

Put the buckwheat in a pot with 500 ml of water, a pinch of salt, and bring to a boil. Cover and cook for 10 minutes, then turn off and let cool with the lid on. Add the spices, garlic, and a part of the breadcrumbs; form flattened meatballs, bread them and fry them in boiling oil. Chop and sauté the onion with a little water and oil for about 8-10 minutes; then add the puree, olives, chopped basil, salt, and pepper. Continue cooking for about 30 minutes. Serve the pancakes hot with the sauce.

14) Rice balls with broccoli and almond pesto

Ingredients:

For the stuffing

• already cooked rice

• extra virgin olive oil or seeds for frying

For the batter

• chickpea flour

• water q.s.

• a pinch of salt

• breadcrumbs

For the broccoli and almond pesto

• half a fresh broccoli

• 80 g of almonds

• the juice of half a lemon

• a clove of garlic

• a large tuft of fresh parsley

• Salt to taste.

• extra virgin olive oil as needed

Let's start by preparing the broccoli and almond pesto. Cut your broccoli

into small pieces and steam it or cook it in a pot in hot water for a maximum of 10 minutes. Put it in the blender and add the remaining ingredients: the garlic clove into small pieces, the parsley, the lemon juice, the almonds, the salt, and the olive oil. Blend vigorously, help yourself using a little water if necessary (the one used for cooking broccoli, for example), taste, and season with salt. Put the pesto in a large bowl and let the ingredients rest. At this point, we proceed with the preparation and cooking of the meatballs. In a bowl, mix the chickpea flour with water, avoiding the formation of lumps. Mix vigorously until you get a thick and homogeneous batter. Add a pinch of salt. Prepare a dish with the center's breadcrumbs: you can make your breading even tastier by adding chopped aromatic herbs, garlic or onion, sesame seeds, or chopped hazelnuts. Take some rice and form a ball with wet hands that you will dip first in the batter and then pass it in the breadcrumbs. Repeat the operation until the dough is used up. Prepare a pot with a high bottom and put the oil to heat. Once the temperature is reached, start frying your meatballs for a few minutes until they are golden and place them in a dish lined with absorbent paper. Take a serving dish, place your hot and crunchy meatballs in the center, bring to the table and serve them accompanied by the broccoli and almond pesto sauce.

15) Fennel in orange cream

Ingredients:

- **2 medium fennel**
- **1 cup of cashews**
- **125 ml of orange juice**
- **2 teaspoons of dried mint**
- **1 pinch of chilli**
- **1 tablespoon of oil**
- **½ teaspoon of salt**
- **1 teaspoon of agave syrup**

Wash the fennel, cut them into four parts, and, using a mandolin, slice them finely. Sprinkle it with salt and let it rest. Meanwhile, prepare the cream. Put the cashews in the blender with the orange juice, mint, chili pepper, oil, salt, and agave syrup and mix until the mixture is fluid and without lumps. Drain the fennel water and season with the cream.

Chapter 5: Soups and salads

1) Oat milk mushroom cream

Ingredients:

- 2 shallots
- 2 tablespoons of flour
- 400 ml of vegetable broth
- 200 ml of oat milk
- 400 g of mushrooms
- 20 g of dried porcini mushrooms
- ½ teaspoon of marjoram
- 1 tablespoon of chopped parsley
- 2 tablespoons of oil
- 100 g of oat flakes
- salt

Rinse the dried mushrooms and soak them in hot water for 30 minutes. Filter the liquid and squeeze the porcini mushrooms, then cut them up. Spread the flakes in a single layer on a baking sheet lined with baking paper, bake them at 180 ° and toast them for 10 minutes, turning them now and then. Let them cool. Meanwhile, you have cleaned the mushrooms with a damp cloth and sliced them. Chop the shallots and put them in a pan with a little broth, marjoram, and a pinch of salt. Let them soften over medium heat, then add the fresh and dried mushrooms. Stir, sprinkle with flour and pour in the hot oat milk without stopping stirring from avoiding lumps. Sprinkle with the rest of the hot broth and the soaking water of the porcini mushrooms. Cook the soup for about 20 minutes, then blend it by immersion. Season it with salt, season it with oil and transfer it to the soup plates, where you have distributed the toasted flakes. Garnish with parsley and serve.

2) Spelled and potato soup

Ingredients:
- **250 g of spelled**
- **3 potatoes**
- **1 red onion**
- **1 heart of celery**
- **2 carrots**
- **100 g of peeled tomatoes**
- **extra virgin olive oil**
- **salt and pepper**

Soak the spelled in cold water overnight. The next day, rinse it and cook it in a pot with one and a half liters of salted water for about 20 minutes. Peel the potatoes and onion, peel the carrot and celery. Cut all the vegetables into cubes or small pieces. In an earthenware pot, first brown a fried onion, celery, and carrots with a salt pinch. Just wilted, add the potatoes and tomatoes. Stew on low heat. Halfway through cooking, pour about a liter of boiling water and continue to cook for 20 minutes. Once cooked, pass the vegetables through a vegetable mill and add the boiled spelled. Mix the ingredients and season with salt and pepper. Serve the soup dressed with raw extra virgin olive oil.

3) Carrot soup with almonds

Ingredients:
- **2 potatoes**
- **1 kg of carrots**
- **500 g of fennel**
- **1 stalk of celery**
- **1 onion**
- **150 g of almonds**
- **1 bunch of parsley**
- **2-3 tablespoons of sunflower oil**

Wash the fennel and celery, peel the onion, potatoes, and carrots; cut the prepared vegetables into small pieces and chop the almonds. Collect everything in a pot. Pour enough water to cover the vegetables by about two fingers. Bring to a boil, reduce the heat; cook for about 30 minutes, remove from heat, and work the mixture with the hand blender until creamy. Season with salt and complete with the washed and chopped parsley and sunflower oil.

4) Pumpkin and cauliflower soup

Ingredients:
- **a small pumpkin**
- **an onion**
- **half a teaspoon of salt**
- **a cup of cauliflower**
- **a teaspoon of white miso**

In a saucepan, arrange the diced onion and diced pumpkin. Cover with water, add salt and cook until the vegetables are well softened. Blend until you get a soft pumpkin cream. In a saucepan of boiling water, cook the pieces of cauliflower for 2-3 minutes. Drain and add them to the pumpkin cream. Dress with white miso. Garnish with parsley and serve.

5)   Cream of purple potatoes

Ingredients:
- **600 g of purple potatoes**
- **200 g of cooked pumpkin**
- **2 onions**
- **1 dl of oat cream**
- **1 stick of celery**
- **1 carrot**
- **200 g baguette**
- **extra virgin olive oil**
- **2 cloves of garlic**
- **salt**

Peel the onions, chop one finely and set it aside. Put the other whole onion in a liter of water and boil for the vegetable broth. We combine the cleaned carrot and celery stalk and let it boil for 40 minutes, then filter and prepare the cream. In a saucepan, put the chopped onion with a little oil; when it is golden, add the purple potatoes, washed, peeled, and diced. After about ten minutes, gradually add the broth, stir and cook over moderate heat for about half an hour. Meanwhile, brown the chopped garlic in a pan with plenty of oil, then remove it and brown the bread cut into cubes of about one centimeter. Pour the cream into the pan with the potatoes, blend everything by immersion, season with salt, and season with oil. We also purée the cooked pumpkin, salt lightly, and let a few small spoonfuls slide over the cream, trying to keep the orange patches spaced apart. Finally, we serve a small bowl accompanied with the croutons to soak.

6) Tasty coleslaw

Ingredients:
- **¼ of white cabbage**
- **¼ of red cabbage**
- **2 carrots**
- **1 teaspoon of brown sugar**
- **1 tablespoon of apple cider vinegar**
- **5 tablespoons of vegan low-fat mayonnaise**
- **1 teaspoon of Dijon mustard**
- **1 piece of onion**

Wash the two types of cabbage, dry them, and cut them very thin. Rinse the carrots and, with the help of a potato peeler, cut them into slices lengthwise. Mix the vegetables, add the salt, sugar, and vinegar. Stir well and transfer to a colander. Let it macerate for an hour. After this time, squeeze the vegetables and place them in a salad bowl. Stir in the chopped onion and mayonnaise mixed with the mustard. Mix well and serve.

7)   Spelled and bean soup

Ingredients:
- **120 g of beans**
- **150 g of pearl spelled**
- **1-2 tablespoons of extra virgin olive oil**
- **1 small leek**
- **2 celery sticks**
- **1 carrot**
- **1 piece of pumpkin**
- **1 potato**
- **about 2 liters of vegetable broth**
- **1 bunch of herbs (sage, rosemary, bay leaf)**
- **1 pinch of red pepper**
- **a small sprig of chopped parsley**
- **1 teaspoon of salt**

Soak the beans for 12 hours; remove the soaking water, cover abundantly with fresh water, bring to a boil; then cook for an hour and a half over low heat, adding salt towards the end of cooking. Take half of the beans with the cooking water and pass them through a vegetable mill. Cut the vegetables into cubes, toss the leek in the oil first for 1-2 minutes and then all the others with the salt and chilli. Add the spelled, the bunch of herbs and the vegetable broth; cook in a covered pot over low heat for 30 minutes. Add the beans (pureed and whole), and continue cooking for another 15 minutes. Let the soup rest for about an hour before serving (but it is also good right away!), Garnish each portion with a drizzle of oil and chopped parsley.

8) Cream of barley

Ingredients:
- **300 g of barley**
- **2 l of vegetable broth**
- **1 sprig of rosemary**
- **1 clove of garlic**
- **2 carrots**
- **2 sticks of celery with the leaves**
- **1 onion**
- **1 kohlrabi with leaves**
- **6 sprigs of parsley**
- **4 tablespoons of soy cream**
- **2 teaspoons of turmeric**

Soak the barley overnight, then drain and rinse it. Boil the broth with garlic and rosemary without the sprig. Add the barley, lower the heat and cook for 30 minutes. Meanwhile, clean the carrots, celery, onion, and kohlrabi. Cut them into small pieces and add them to the barley. Season with turmeric and pepper. Continue cooking for about 20 minutes. Finally, pass everything to the mixer. Add the soy cream and heat the cream over low heat. Season with salt and serve.

9)   Colorful buckwheat salad

Ingredients:
- **300 g of buckwheat**
- **2 bay leaves**
- **250 g of boiled green beans**
- **4 ripe tomatoes**
- **1 large bunch of fresh basil**
- **100 g of green olives**
- **1 small clove of garlic**
- **200 g of canned corn**
- **oil**
- **salt and pepper**

Toast the buckwheat without adding fat and cook it with double the water for 20 minutes: when it boils, lower the heat and cook covered with salt and bay leaf. Drain it and let it cool. Meanwhile, wash the tomatoes and green beans, remove the seeds from the first and chop with the second. Rinse the basil well and blend it with the pitted olives, the chopped garlic in quarters, pepper, salt, and oil. Spread the dressing over the cereal, mix the other ingredients and serve this salad cold.

10) Coconut vegetable stew

Ingredients:
- 1 tablespoon of oil
- 1 medium white onion
- 2 cloves of garlic
- 1 fresh hot red pepper
- 400 g of tomatoes
- 200 g of green beans
- 250 g of cooked black beans
- 2 potatoes
- 400 ml of coconut milk
- the juice of 1 lime
- 1 handful of fresh coriander
- 2 handfuls of roasted cashews, lightly salted
- salt
- water
- cooked rice (optional)

Heat the oil over high heat in a thick-bottomed saucepan. Brown the peeled and chopped onion, add the cleaned and chopped garlic and chili pepper, the peeled and diced tomatoes and potatoes, add salt and leave to flavor briefly, stirring constantly. Lower the heat, stir in the sprouted and chopped green beans, and if necessary, pour a little water, cover, and continue cooking for 5-10 minutes. When the potatoes are tender enough, add the black beans and coconut milk and cook. Once you have reached the consistency of a soft stew, remove from heat, sprinkle with lime juice, season with salt, mix and divide into plates. Complete with cashews and coriander washed and fragmented; serve with rice.

11) Fresh barley salad

Ingredients:
- **300 g of barley**
- **800 ml of vegetable broth**
- **1 cucumber**
- **3 medium ripe tomatoes**
- **2 sweet green chillies**
- **10 champignon mushrooms**
- **1 shallot**
- **1 small bunch of basil**
- **1 clove of garlic**
- **2 tablespoons of sunflower seeds**
- **the juice of 1 lemon**
- **4 tablespoons of oil, salt**

Soak the barley overnight. Rinse it and transfer it to a saucepan with the cold broth. Cover and boil it, lower the heat and cook for 40-50 minutes until the liquid runs out. Season the barley with a tablespoon of oil and let it cool. Clean the peppers, cucumber, and tomatoes. Cut the first into rings, the second into cubes, and the third into slices. Put them in a salad bowl. Add the salt and lemon juice. Clean and slice the mushrooms. Add them to the salad along with the finely chopped shallots. Wash the basil, dry it and transfer it to the mixer with the rest of the oil, garlic, and sunflower seeds. Work until you get a homogeneous mixture, helping yourself if needed with a little water. Mix everything with the barley, turn well and let it rest in the fridge for an hour. Serve at room temperature.

12) Peach, parmesan and rocket salad

Ingredients:
- 2 yellow peaches
- 80 g of rocket
- 80 g parmesan
- 7-8 tablespoons of extra virgin olive oil
- 3 teaspoons of black sesame seeds
- salt

Divide the peaches in half, remove the stone and peel them (if they are too ripe, peel them before halving and peeling them); then slice them thinly. Arrange the washed and dried rocket on four plates; distribute the prepared fruits and season the salad with oil and a light sprinkling of salt. Ultimate by distributing in each portion the pecorino reduced to flakes and sesame seeds.

13) Cold avocado soup

Ingredients:
- 1 handful of fresh coriander
- 1 clove of garlic
- a few tufts of chives
- the juice of 1 lime
- a few pinches of cumin powder
- a few pinches of nutmeg
- salt
- black pepper

Combine the peeled and pitted avocados, the peeled and chopped garlic, the cleaned and chopped chives, the lime, the cumin, the nutmeg, salt, and pepper in a blender. Blend, adding cold water in small quantities until you reach a soft consistency. Add the washed and chopped coriander, work the mixture again to mix it, and transfer it to a bowl. Put it in the refrigerator to cool. Serve it in individual bowls, completing, if you like, with a little cream and a few leaves of fresh coriander or chopped chives.

14) Onion soup

Ingredients:
- **800 g of red onions**
- **1 l of vegetable broth**
- **2 medium potatoes**
- **2 tablespoons of oil**
- **salt**
- **1 chilli or 1 clove of garlic**
- **2 slices of stale wholemeal bread**
- **1 tablespoon of cheese**

Peel the onions and slice them thinly. Put them in the cooking pan with the peeled, washed, and diced potatoes. Cover with the cold broth and boil. Lower the heat and keep the pot slightly uncovered. Cook for about 40 minutes. In the end, the onions should be nice and creamy. Season with salt and season with oil. Rub the slices of bread with chili or garlic and arrange them on the bottom of the bowls. Cover with the soup, sprinkle with cheese, and serve immediately.

15) Cream of spinach with pine nuts

Ingredients:
- 1 kg of spinach
- 2 shallots
- 500 ml of vegetable broth
- 100 ml of soy milk
- 100 g of creamy tofu
- 2 tablespoons of flour
- 2 tablespoons of pine nuts
- 2 teaspoons of turmeric
- 2 tablespoons of oil
- salt and pepper

Clean the spinach, wash and drain them. Finely chop the shallots and let them soften in a saucepan with a little broth for about ten minutes. Add the flour, stir to avoid lumps, and add the spinach. Add salt, stir briefly and pour in the warmed milk and remaining broth, tofu, and turmeric. Cook for about ten minutes and blend by immersion. Peppered, seasoned with oil, and served garnished with lightly toasted pine nuts and, if desired, with oat cakes.

Chapter 6: Single course

1) Lentil and rice pie

Ingredients:
- **200 g of lentils**
- **250 g of rice**
- **vegetable broth**
- **2 shallots**
- **2 carrots**
- **1 medium potato**
- **500 g of celeriac**
- **1 bay leaf**
- **3 tablespoons of oil**
- **2 tablespoons of tamari**
- **bread crumbs**
- **3 tablespoons of sesame**
- **1 teaspoon of paprika**
- **1 teaspoon of oregano**
- **salt and chilli**

Soak the lentils for a few hours, drain and boil them for about 40 minutes in water with the bay leaf. Salt towards the end. Gather the rice and 600 ml of broth in a saucepan. With the lid on, boil and reduce the heat. Cook until the liquid runs out. Finely chop the shallots and place them in a pan with oregano, chili, and paprika. Salt and add enough water to cover flush. Cook over medium heat, stirring occasionally. After a few minutes, add the potato, carrots, and celeriac cut into cubes. Stir and pour in a little hot broth. Stew over low heat, adding more hot broth when needed. In the end, transfer the vegetables to the mixer to obtain a thick and creamy mixture, helping you in the case with a little broth. Grease a mold with a bit of oil where you transfer the rice mixed with the lentils. Drizzle with the remaining oil and soy sauce. Cover with vegetable cream and sprinkle with breadcrumbs mixed with sesame. Bake at 180 degrees for about 20 minutes. Serve the pie hot.

2) Ricotta and walnut pie

Ingredients:
- **500 g of ricotta**
- **4-5 tablespoons of lightly toasted walnuts**
- **2 tablespoons of milk**
- **4 nice pinches of saffron stigmas**
- **3 tablespoons of marjoram leaves**
- **salt**
- **oil for the molds**

Infuse the saffron in hot milk for about an hour. Pour the infusion over the ricotta you have sifted into a bowl, add the coarsely chopped walnuts and marjoram, season with salt. Mix all the ingredients to form a cream that you will distribute in the individual round casseroles about 10-12 centimeters wide, greased with a drizzle of oil. Bake for 20 minutes at 180 degrees. When the patties are ready, take them out of the oven and gently remove them from the molds; arrange them in the center of the plates, accompanying them with salads arranged in a crown and possibly dressed with a light vinaigrette.

3)   White bean paté with caper pesto

Ingredients:
- **300 g cannellini beans (cooked weight)**
- **30 g of onion**
- **30 g of Evo oil**
- **20 g of salted capers**
- **15 g of lemon juice**
- **10 g of lemon zest**
- **a bay leaf**

Boil the beans, which you have previously soaked for at least 12 hours, with a bay leaf. Soak the capers in plenty of warm water and leave them to desalt for the entire preparation time. Then reduce them to a puree, mashing them with a fork or blending them with a hand blender. Help yourself with half the oil and lemon juice to make the pate more homogeneous and fluffy. Separately, chop the onion and cut the lemon zest into thin strips. Drain the capers and chop them coarsely. Place the pate on a plate, season it with the remaining extra virgin olive oil, onion, lemon peel, and capers. Serve at the table cold or room temperature, accompanied by slices of toasted bread.

4) Chickpea stew

Ingredients:
- **a cup of chickpeas left to soak overnight**
- **2 teaspoons of extra virgin olive oil**
- **2 onions**
- **2 carrots**
- **2 cloves of garlic**
- **2 celery sticks**
- **2 bay leaves**
- **2-3 tablespoons of miso**

Drain the chickpeas and cook them in a pot full of water for about an hour over medium heat. Cut the vegetables and brown them in a pan with oil for about 5 minutes over high heat. Add the vegetables and bay leaves to the beans and simmer until the vegetables are well cooked. Add the miso and cook for a few more minutes. Serve with a sprinkling of chopped parsley.

5) Pasta and cauliflower

Ingredients:
- **350 g of wholemeal short pasta**
- **1 cauliflower of 800 g**
- **400 g of peeled tomatoes**
- **3 tablespoons of oil**
- **2 cloves of garlic**
- **1 teaspoon of marjoram**
- **1 teaspoon of spicy paprika**
- **50 g of Parmesan cheese**

Clean the cauliflower, wash it, divide it into florets and steam it for 10-15 minutes. Meanwhile, put the crushed tomatoes with a fork, chopped garlic, marjoram, paprika, salt in a saucepan. Cook them for about 15 minutes. Add the cauliflower. Cook for a few minutes, stirring. Bring water to boil in a saucepan. When it comes to the boil, cook the pasta for the time indicated on the package. Drain and pour the cauliflower pasta. Grate the cheese, turn the heat back on under the pasta and stir for 1 minute over medium heat. Season with oil, season with salt, and serve.

6)   Eggplant stuffed with mushrooms

Ingredients:
- **4 medium eggplants**
- **300 g of champignon mushrooms**
- **1 red onion**
- **1 clove of garlic**
- **100 g of tomato sauce**
- **1 small bunch of fresh thyme**
- **bread crumbs**
- **3 tablespoons of oil, salt**

Wash and clean the eggplants, dry them and divide them in half lengthwise. Dig them inside with a sharp knife, being careful not to break the shell. Cut the pulp into cubes and cook in a pan where you have done withered the onion with a little water. Add salt, stir for a few minutes over medium heat and add the puree. Cook for 10 minutes. Clean and slice the mushrooms. Stew them in a pan with the peeled and halved garlic and 1 tablespoon of oil. After 15 minutes on low heat, turn off and add salt. Mix the mushrooms with the eggplant pulp and season with the remaining oil. Season with salt and complete with chopped thyme. Fill the eggplants with this mixture and sprinkle them with breadcrumbs. Arrange them on a baking sheet lined with parchment paper and bake at 190 ° for 40-50 minutes. Serve warm or hot.

7)   Rice salad in tomatoes

Ingredients:
- **4 large ripe but firm tomatoes**
- **200 g of brown rice**
- **500 ml of broth**
- **1 spring onion**
- **80 g of mayonnaise)**
- **10 pitted green olives**
- **a few sprigs of fresh marjoram**
- **salt**

Pour the rice and broth into a saucepan. Put the lid on; when it boils, lower the heat and cook for 40-45 minutes. In the last 10 minutes add the green part of the onion, washed and shredded. When cooked, add salt to the rice and let it cool. Wash the tomatoes, remove the top cap, empty them internally and add salt. Mix the mayonnaise with the rice; if the mixture is too dry, add a little tomato pulp (saving the rest for a salad or a sauce). Incorporate a mixture made with the white onion and marjoram. Complete with the chopped olives and stuff the tomatoes with the mixture obtained. Cover them with the cap and let them rest in the fridge for half an hour before serving.

8)   Pasta with cherry tomatoes and capers

Ingredients:
- **280 g of wholemeal pasta of your choice**
- **12-15 cherry tomatoes, cleaned and quartered**
- **4-5 tablespoons of extra virgin olive oil**
- **half a white onion, peeled and chopped**
- **2 spicy green peppers, cleaned and chopped**
- **1 generous handful of salted capers**
- **1 handful of fresh, clean oregano**

Soak the capers in cold water for about 20 minutes, rinse and drain. Cook the pasta in abundant salted water. Meanwhile, heat the oil in a large pan and lightly soften the onion. Add the chilies, tomatoes and cook the capers for 4-5 minutes beforehand. Once the pasta is cooked, drain and add it to the sauce. Stir a couple of minutes, remove from heat, stir and serve.

9)   Zucchini stuffed with chickpeas

Ingredients:
- 4 medium-large zucchini
- vegetable broth q.s.
- 250 g of boiled chickpeas
- 2 shallots
- 1 teaspoon of coriander seeds
- 20 g of dried mushrooms
- 1 teaspoon of marjoram
- the juice of 1/2 lemon
- 3 tablespoons of oil
- Salt to taste

Soak the mushrooms in warm water for 30 minutes. Wash the zucchini and steam them whole for 5 minutes. Let them cool, tick them, and cut them in half lengthwise; gently dig them to remove most of the pulp, taking care not to break the peel. Set them aside. Finely chop the shallots and let them soften for a few minutes in a pan, lightly covered with broth. Add the marjoram and the squeezed and thinly sliced mushrooms. Follow with the crushed coriander and salt. Cook for 10 minutes on low heat, finally adds the chickpeas, a tablespoon of oil, and lemon juice. Stir and turn off the heat. Blend by immersion, helping you if needed with a little broth but trying to keep the mixture firm. Transfer it to the zucchini shells, which you will then line up on a baking sheet lined with baking paper. Bake at 180 degrees for about 30 minutes. Serve the dish hot or warm, seasoned with the remaining oil.

10) Rice and peas

Ingredients:
- **200 g of rice**
- **1 Kg of peas**
- **garlic**
- **parsley**
- **extra virgin olive oil**
- **salt and pepper**

Bring salted water to a boil for cooking the rice. Meanwhile, in a pan, cook the shelled peas cold with finely chopped garlic and parsley and a glass of water. When almost cooked, evaporate any excess water, add salt, and season with extra virgin olive oil. Serve the boiled rice with the peas.

11) Pasta with chickpeas and celery pesto

Ingredients:
- **250 g of pasta**
- **150 g of cooked chickpeas**
- **70 g of tender ribs and celery leaves**
- **50 g of linseed or sesame seeds**
- **50 ml of water from pasta or legumes**
- **oil and salt**

Prepare the pesto. Lightly toast the flax (or sesame) seeds in a non-stick pan. After a couple of minutes, turn off the heat. Peel the celery and wash it, dry it and chop it. Put it in the hand blender's jar with the seeds and water from the pasta (or chickpeas). Add lightly salt and stir, gradually adding the oil needed to obtain a soft cream, similar to cream. In the meantime, you will have boiled the pasta al dente. Drain it, mix it with the chickpeas and season with the celery pesto, then serve it.

12) Spaghetti with walnut and basil sauce

Ingredients:
- **400 g of spaghetti**
- **100 g of shelled walnuts**
- **80 g of pine nuts**
- **1 clove of garlic**
- **30 g of basil leaves**
- **2 tablespoons of grated pecorino**
- **3 tablespoons of oil**
- **salt**

Prepare the sauce. Spread the walnuts and half of the pine nuts on a baking tray in a single layer. Bake them at 150 ° for about ten minutes until they are lightly toasted. During this time, stir them a couple of times. Let them cool down and remove the skin by rubbing them. Put them in a mixer with a little salt and chop finely. Add the peeled and chopped garlic, then washed and dried basil, a few tablespoons of hot water. Continue to work the ingredients until they are homogeneous, adding a little more hot water. Complete with oil. Cook the spaghetti in boiling salted water, drain when al dente, and season immediately with the walnut and basil sauce. Sprinkle them with the grated Parmesan and serve.

13) Spelled and pistachio flans with carrot and tofu cream

Ingredients:
For the flans:

- 350 g of spelled
- 850 ml of water
- 250 g of shelled pistachios
- 5 tablespoons of extra virgin olive oil
- a bunch of basil
- 1 clove of garlic
- 150 ml of soy cream
- salt and pepper

For the carrot and tofu cream:
- 250 g of fresh tofu
- 250 g of carrots
- 150 ml of soy milk
- 3 tablespoons of sunflower oil
- 2 teaspoons of lemon juice
- 1 teaspoon of paprika and salt

For the pesto, remove the skin from the pistachios by immersing them for a couple of minutes in boiling water. Grind them in the mixer for 1 minute with the oil, the washed and dried basil, and the peeled garlic. Add the cream, salt, pepper, and operate for another minute. Wash the spelled, drain it, and put it in a saucepan with salted water. Bring to a boil and reduce the heat to low. Cover and continue cooking without stirring for 35-40 minutes. Finally, add the pistachio pesto. Meanwhile, prepare the carrot and tofu cream. Boil the tofu for about 10 minutes in lightly salted water with the peeled and chopped carrots. Drain them and put them in a mixer with the sunflower oil, salt, lemon juice, and paprika; operate and add the soy milk a little at a time until it forms a soft and smooth cream. Oil the molds and fill them with spelled pressing them well with a spoon, let them rest for a few minutes. Bake the flans in the oven at 180 degrees for 40 minutes. Turn the flans over onto serving plates, cover with a couple of tablespoons of cream and serve.

14) Artichoke and lentil cake pan

Ingredients:
- **12 artichokes**
- **1 lemon**
- **300 g of lentils**
- **2 shallots**
- **1 sprig of rosemary**
- **1 sprig of sage**
- **1 teaspoon of thyme**
- **vegetable broth**
- **bread crumbs**
- **4 tablespoons of oil**
- **salt**

Soak the lentils overnight, rinse them and place them in a saucepan with the chopped rosemary and sage. Cover them with cold water and cook for about 40 minutes. Add salt only at the end. Clean the artichokes, halve them and wash them in water acidulated with lemon juice. Cook them al dente in a pan with the thyme, a tablespoon of oil, and a little water, salt. Be careful not to break them and keep them crunchy. Blend the lentils until the mixture is not too moist. Finely chop the shallots, let them dry in a pan with a tablespoon of oil and a little water. Add the past and let it flavor for a few minutes. Add another tablespoon of oil and stir. Grease a round mold with high sides, and sprinkle it with breadcrumbs. Form the first layer with half of the artichokes. Pour half of the remaining oil, distribute the legume purée and arrange the rest of the artichokes on the surface. Season with the remaining oil and bake at 190 ° for 10 minutes. Serve the dish hot.

15) Brown rice with ginger

Ingredients:
- **400 g of cooked brown rice**
- **2 spring onions**
- **1 carrot**
- **cabbage 350 g**
- **2 tablespoons of oil**
- **salt**
- **1 piece of ginger root**

Cut the spring onions into rings, the carrot into not too thin matches, and the cabbage into strips. Grease a pan with oil and toss the spring onions with a pinch of salt for a minute. Then add the carrot, cabbage, and another pinch of salt and sauté for another 8-9 minutes, often stirring, until the vegetables begin to be tender (possibly add a couple of tablespoons of water). Then add the cooked rice and a little water to the pan's bottom, cook covered for 5 minutes. Finally, season with the ginger juice, mix, and serve.

Chapter 7: Fish

1) Crispy salmon

Ingredients:
- **Salmon fillet (4 of 250 g each) 1 kg**
- **Bread 100 g**
- **1 sprig parsley**
- **Dill 1 sprig**
- **Thyme 4 sprigs**
- **Rosemary 2 sprigs**
- **Lemon zest 1**
- **Extra virgin olive oil 50 g**
- **White pepper in grains 1 tsp**
- **Salt up to taste**

First, prepare the breading: cut the bread into pieces and put it in a mixer, then add the dill, the peeled thyme, the needles of rosemary and parsley. Pour in the oil too, then add the lemon zest, salt and white pepper. Blend until you get a coarse consistency. Now take care of the salmon fillets: remove the skin with a thin-bladed knife and remove the bones with the help of a kitchen tongs, then transfer the fillets to a drip pan lined with parchment paper and cover them with the breading, making it adhere well with your hands. . After covering the fillets evenly, cook in a preheated convection oven at 190 ° for about 20 minutes. After the cooking time, take out and serve your crispy salmon hot!

2) Baked salmon

Ingredients:
- **Salmon steaks (4 pieces) 660 g**
- **Potatoes 170 g**
- **Lemon zest 1**
- **Lemon juice 25 g**
- **Dry white wine 25 g**
- **Extra virgin olive oil 50 g**
- **Parsley to chop 1 tbsp**
- **Salt up to taste**
- **Black pepper to taste**

To prepare the baked salmon, first remove the fish bones with tweezers and check that there are no bones left by sliding a fingertip on the pulp. Remove the spine with a knife, then roll one end on itself and wrap the other end around the slice to obtain a medallion. Tie the medallion with a kitchen string to ensure that it maintains the shape even during cooking and transfer the medallions on a baking sheet lined with parchment paper. Take a fairly regular shaped potato, wash it and cut it into thin slices with a mandolin, without peeling it: the slices must be no more than 1 mm thick otherwise they will not be cooked enough. Now take care of the emulsion: grate the zest of a lemon in a bowl, then add 25 g of lemon juice, oil, white wine, chopped parsley, salt and pepper and mix well with a fork. Season the salmon medallions with part of the emulsion, then cover them with the slightly overlapping potato discs and sprinkle the potatoes with the remaining emulsion. When the medallions are ready, bake in a preheated static oven at 180 ° for about 20 minutes, then operate the grill at 240 ° and continue cooking for another 3-4 minutes, until the potatoes are golden. After the cooking time has elapsed, remove the cooking string and immediately serve your delicious baked salmon!

3)   Salmon rice

Ingredients:
•Rice 350 g
•Salmon steaks 250 g
•Leeks 1
•Extra virgin olive oil q.s.
•1 clove garlic
•½ glass white wine
•Parmesan to be grated 20 g
•Salt up to taste
•Black pepper to taste
•Fish broth 500 ml

FOR THE FLAVORED BUTTER
•Butter 80 g
•Marjoram 1 sprig
•Dill 1 sprig
•Thyme 1 sprig
•Lemon zest ½
•Salt up to taste

Prepare the flavored butter by chopping the herbs and grating the lemon zest, allow the butter to soften at room temperature and when it has reached a creamy consistency add the chopped herbs, lemon zest and salt. Meanwhile, clean the salmon steak and cut it into small pieces. Heat a tablespoon of oil in a pan with a clove of whole garlic and brown the salmon bites for 2/3 minutes, add salt and set the salmon aside, removing the garlic. Now start preparing the risotto: finely chop the leek and sauté it over low heat with two tablespoons of oil in a pan. Pour in the rice and toast it for a few moments over high heat, stirring with a wooden spoon. Deglaze with the counter wine and continue cooking, stirring occasionally, taking care that the rice does not stick, adding the broth (vegetable or fish) a little at a time. Halfway through cooking add the salmon morsels, season with salt if necessary and when the rice is well cooked, remove it from the heat and stir in the herb-flavored butter and a couple of tablespoons of grated cheese, if you like.

4) Mediterranean-style salmon fillets

Ingredients:
- **Salmon 800 g**
- **Cherry tomatoes 350 g**
- **Dried oregano 1 sprig**
- **Extra virgin olive oil 30 g**
- **Salt up to taste**
- **1 clove garlic**
- **Pitted black olives 70 g**
- **Pickled capers 5 g**

Start washing the tomatoes, then dry them and cut them into 4. Transfer them to a large bowl, add the peeled and halved garlic and the chopped dried oregano. Add the oil, salt, mix everything and cover with cling film. Let the tomatoes macerate for about 1 hour at room temperature. After this time, take the salmon steak and remove any bones with tweezers and remove the skin if it is present; then cut into 4 fillets of equal thickness. Take back the cherry tomatoes, remove the garlic and transfer them to a lightly greased baking dish. Arrange the salmon fillets on top of the cherry tomatoes and with a teaspoon take some cherry tomatoes and arrange them on top of the salmon. Salt, pepper, add the black olives and capers. Bake in a preheated static oven at 180 ° for about 15 minutes (if you want to use the convection oven, bake at 160 ° for about 10 minutes). After this time, take out and serve your Mediterranean salmon fillets still hot!

5) Tuna tartare

Ingredients:
- **Tuna in slices 450 g**
- **Oranges 1**
- **Extra virgin olive oil 40 g**
- **Salt up to taste**
- **Black pepper to taste**
- **Shortcrust pastry 230 g**
- **Wild fennel 3 sprigs**

Start grating the zest of an orange, then cut it in half and squeeze the juice. In a bowl, pour the extra virgin olive oil, the orange juice and its zest. Finely chop the fennel, keeping a few strands aside for the final decoration, add it to the mixture and emulsify with a whisk. Meanwhile, prepare the shortcrust pastry shells. Adjust the emulsion with a pinch of pepper and salt. Prepare the shortcrust pastry shells that will be used to make tartare single portions: roll out the shortcrust pastry (you can use a roll of already made shortcrust pastry), cut out 10 circles of about 10 cm in diameter and line 10 round molds with a diameter of 8 cm , after having buttered them. Prick the bottom with the tines of a fork and cook in white, covered with dried legumes as weight, in the oven at 180 degrees for 10-15 minutes. When they are golden, take them out of the oven, let them cool and turn them out. Take the tuna steaks: make sure you have bought especially fish. It is recommended to freeze it for 96 hours at -18 degrees and then defrost it for use in the recipe. Rinse and dry the tuna fillets with absorbent paper. Cut them into small cubes half a centimeter thick and place them in a large bowl. Pour the oil and orange emulsion over them and mix so that the tuna is well flavored. Then fill the cakes with one or two tablespoons of tuna tartare and decorate your tartare with a few sprigs of fennel.

6) Tuna in pistachio crust

Ingredients:
- **Tuna 600 g**
- **Poppy seeds 1 tbsp**
- **Extra virgin olive oil 3 tbsp**
- **Breadcrumbs 20 g**
- **Chopped pistachios 50**
- **Dried tomatoes in oil 30 g**
- **Salt up to taste**

Get yourself a slice of fresh tuna, place the slice in the freezer for at least an hour so that it is more convenient to cut without breaking the fibers. Remove the tuna from the freezer and cut it lengthwise into slices about 2-3 cm thick. Put the tuna slices in a baking dish and drizzle them with the olive oil. Meanwhile, dry the dried tomatoes with a cloth to remove excess oil and chop finely with a knife. Place the chopped pistachios in a bowl, add the chopped tomatoes, poppy seeds and breadcrumbs. Stir to mix the ingredients well and salt the breading to taste. Take the slices of tuna and pass them in the breadcrumbs, pressing well on all sides. Place a couple of tablespoons of extra virgin olive oil in a non-stick pan and once the necessary heat is reached, add the breaded tuna slices and cook them for 1 minute per side, turning them only once. Do not continue cooking so that the tuna remains pink inside, the tuna must not turn white otherwise the meat will be harder. Remove the pistachio crusted tuna from the pan and cut into 2 cm thick slices, then place them on a serving dish and serve immediately.

7)   Spaghetti with tuna

Ingredients:
- **Spaghetti 320 g**
- **Tuna in oil (drained) 150 g**
- **Peeled tomatoes 400 g**
- **Extra virgin olive oil q.s.**
- **Salt up to taste**
- **Black pepper to taste**
- **Basil to taste**
- **Onions ½**

Start by putting a pot full of water on the stove, add salt to taste when boiling: it will be used for cooking the pasta. Drain the tuna fillet from the conservation oil. Meanwhile, peel the onion, slice it thinly. Heat the olive oil in a pan and add the sliced onion. Let it dry over low heat for a few minutes, stirring often; fray the tuna with your hands and add it to the pan when the onion is soft and let it brown for a couple of minutes, stirring constantly. Now, mash the tomatoes with a fork and pour them into the pan with the tuna; let the sauce cook for about 10 minutes. Meanwhile, cook the spaghetti, while the pasta is cooking, the sauce will also be ready. Drain the spaghetti directly into the pan with the tuna, season with the ground pepper, turn off the heat and perfume with the fresh basil leaves. Stir and serve your tuna spaghetti hot!

8)   Tuna glazed with soy sauce

Ingredients:
- **Tuna fillet 400 g**
- **Red cabbage 500 g**
- **Soy sauce 50 g**
- **White wine vinegar 100 g**
- **Salt up to 30 g**
- **Extra virgin olive oil 20 g**
- **Basil 4 leaves**
- **Sesame seeds 30 g**

Start with the vegetables: julienne the cabbage and place it in a bowl, sprinkling with white wine vinegar and seasoning with salt. Mix the ingredients well and leave to macerate for at least 1 hour, covering with cling film. After this time, drain and rinse the cabbage thoroughly under plenty of running water. Then cook it in a non-stick pan in which you have heated 15 g of oil. Flavored with well washed and dried basil leaves and cover with a lid, cooking over low heat for about 10 minutes. When cooked, the cabbage should still be crunchy. While the cabbage is cooking, dedicate yourself to the tuna. Take a small bowl and pour the soy sauce. Take care of the tuna: make sure you have a fillet already cut down; we advise you to freeze the fillet for at least 96 hours at -18 degrees and then defrost for preparation. Cut the tuna into slices about 4 cm thick. Then place a small bowl next to the soy sauce in which you will have poured the white sesame seeds. Take a slice of tuna and wet it on all sides with the soy sauce, then completely cover the long sides of the tuna slice with sesame seeds. Repeat the operation with all the slices of tuna. Now take a non-stick pan and pour in 5 g of oil: heat it up and place the slices of tuna on the long sides. Blanch the tuna slices for about 2 minutes, then flip them to cook them on the other side for another 2 minutes. For even cooking, you can also sear the tuna slices sideways, 1 minute on each side. Place a bed of cabbage on the serving dish and arrange the slices of tuna on top of it, accompanying with the soy sauce. Your tuna glazed with soy sauce is then ready to be brought to the table and enjoyed!

9) Baked sardines

Ingredients:
- 18 sardines for a total of about 250 g
- Breadcrumbs 60 g
- Extra virgin olive oil 60 g
- 1 sprig parsley
- Thyme 1 sprig
- 1 clove garlic
- Grated Parmesan cheese 20 g
- Pine nuts 30 g
- Extra virgin olive oil to grease the pan 15g

Pour the breadcrumbs, grated cheese and the crushed garlic clove into a bowl. Rinse, dry and finely chop the parsley; then also add it to the breading and further flavor with the thyme leaves; pour the 60 g of oil and mix everything until you get a uniform mixture. At this point take a baking dish measuring 19x15 cm and sprinkle it with about 15 g of oil. Arrange the sardines horizontally without overlapping each other, salt (not excessively), pepper and cover with half of the previously prepared mixture. Arrange another layer of sardines, taking care to position them vertically (opposite to before), salt, pepper and cover the entire surface with the remaining part of the breading. Finish by decorating the surface with pine nuts. Then cook the sardines in the oven in grill mode at 200 ° for 8 minutes, until they are golden brown. Once cooked, serve the baked sardines while still hot.

10) Spaghetti with anchovies and breadcrumbs

Ingredients:
- **Spaghetti 320 g**
- **Anchovies in oil 30 g**
- **Extra virgin olive oil 20 g**
- **Breadcrumbs 70 g**
- **3 cloves garlic**

Put a pan with water on the heat and bring to a boil: it will then be used to cook the pasta. Meanwhile, pour 10 g of extra virgin olive oil into a pan, then add the peeled garlic cloves and the anchovy fillets drained from the preservation oil. Peel a ladle of hot water and pour it into the pan, so you can melt the anchovies in the best possible way. This will take about 10 minutes so stir often. Meanwhile, in a separate pan pour 10 g of extra virgin olive oil, then add breadcrumbs to toast it and mix everything until the crumbs are golden; keep aside. At this point, cook the pasta in boiling water; you can add at most very little coarse salt if you prefer, as anchovies are very tasty. Cook the spaghetti for the time indicated on the package. After the time has elapsed, remove the garlic cloves from the saucepan and drain the pasta by dipping it directly into the pan. Add some of the breadcrumbs and mix. If necessary, add a little more cooking water, then serve your spaghetti with the anchovies and garnish with a final sprinkling of breadcrumbs.

11) Orange mackerel

Ingredients:
•Mackerel (4 whole clean) 1200 g
•Orange peel 1
•Extra virgin olive oil q.s.
FOR MARINATING
•Orange juice
•Extra virgin olive oil 30 g
•Dill 2 sprigs
•2 cloves garlic
•Black peppercorns 1 tbsp
•Salt up to 1 tbsp

Make diagonal cuts on the sides of the mackerel and set aside. Take care of the ingredients for the marinade: with the back of the spoon, crush the peppercorns so they will release their aroma better, then squeeze the juice from the oranges. Peel and thinly slice the garlic. Grease a baking dish with oil, place the mackerel on top and season them on the surface with another drizzle of oil, the peppercorns, salt, scented with the sprigs of dill and flavored with the slices of garlic. Finally, sprinkle the fish with half of the orange juice, cover with plastic wrap and leave to marinate for 2 hours in the refrigerator. After the marinating time, go to cooking: heat a pan with a drizzle of olive oil and, when it is hot, lay the fillets. Let them cook over high heat for 4 minutes without touching them, then turn them, sprinkle them with the remaining orange juice and continue cooking for another 2 minutes. Once the sauce has congealed and the mackerel are well flavored, serve them immediately garnishing them with grated orange zest on the surface.

12) Mackerel in foil

Ingredients:
- **Mackerel (2 clean mackerel)**
- **Celery 90 g**
- **Yellow peppers 70 g**
- **Tomatoes 60 g**
- **Eggplant 50 g**
- **Lemons 1**
- **Basil to taste**
- **Extra virgin olive oil q.s.**
- **Black pepper to taste**
- **Salt up to taste**

Chop the celery and cut it into cubes, then cut the eggplants into slices and cut into cubes. Remove the internal seeds and the stalk of the pepper and cut it first into strips and then into cubes. Finally, cut the tomatoes into cubes. Transfer all the cut vegetables to a bowl, scented with fresh basil leaves and season with oil, salt and pepper. Now place each clean mackerel on a 35x31 cm sheet of parchment paper, fill the belly of the mackerel with a spoonful of vegetables and then distribute the rest around the fish. Season the fish with a drizzle of olive oil. Wash the lemon and cut into thin slices, then place 3 lemon slices on top of each mackerel. Now close the parcel by lifting the flaps of parchment paper and placing them on top of the fish, then seal well by folding the sides. Place the packets on a baking tray lined with parchment paper and bake in a preheated static oven at 200 ° for 20 minutes. When cooked, take your mackerel in foil out of the oven and serve hot.

13) Swordfish with tomato sauce

Ingredients:
- Swordfish (2 slices) 400 g
- Lemons 1
- Marjoram 3 sprigs
- Extra virgin olive oil 30 g
- Salt up to taste
- Black pepper to taste

FOR THE TOMATO SAUCE
- Tomatoes 250 g
- Worcestershire sauce 20 ml
- 1 clove garlic
- Extra virgin olive oil 15 g
- Salt up to taste
- Black pepper to taste

First, take care of the marinade: place the swordfish fillet in a fairly large baking dish, add the oil, the marjoram leaves, the grated rind of a lemon (keep some aside for the final garnish) and the juice. of half a lemon. Turn the fish on both sides to make sure it is evenly flavored, then cover the dish with cling film and set it aside temporarily. Wash the cherry tomatoes and cut them in half; Heat the oil in a pan, add the garlic clove and let it brown briefly. Add the cherry tomatoes, salt, pepper and mix. Then deglaze with the Worcestershire sauce. Let the cherry tomatoes cook for 10 minutes over medium heat, stirring occasionally. Once cooked, turn off the heat, remove the garlic and transfer them to a tall, narrow container, then blend them with an immersion blender until you get a smooth and homogeneous sauce. Heat another pan well, remove the swordfish from the marinade and place it in the pan, add salt and sear the fish over medium-high heat for 2 minutes on one side and for 1 minute on the other. Once cooked, transfer the swordfish to a plate and cut into cubes. At this point you can assemble the serving dishes: sprinkle the bottom with a little tomato sauce, add the swordfish morsels and finally garnish with a few leaves of marjoram, the lemon zest that you had kept aside and a minced pepper: your swordfish with tomato sauce is ready to be served!

14) Swordfish carpaccio with green and pink pepper

Ingredients:
•**Swordfish 500**
•**Semi-skimmed milk 250 g**
•**Pink peppercorns 5**
•**Green peppercorns 10**
•**Extra virgin olive oil 50 g**
•**Himalayan salt (pink) 5 g**

Start by cutting the swordfish slices. Cut the swordfish steak into 16 slices of about 30 g each and 3-4 mm thick. To facilitate the operation, keep the swordfish steak to compact it in the freezer for an hour before slicing it. If you don't have a slicer available, buy the swordfish already cut into slices for the carpaccio or have it cut in your trusted fish shop. Remove the skin of the swordfish with a knife and arrange the slices in a baking dish. Start preparing the marinade: pour the milk and oil into a bowl. Add the green peppercorns, pink pepper and pink Himalayan salt. Emulsify the mixture with a whisk to mix all the ingredients. Pour the marinade into the pan where you have placed the swordfish slices and cover with plastic wrap. The carpaccio must marinate in the refrigerator for at least 4 hours. After this time, remove the swordfish carpaccio from the fridge and, with the help of a spatula, lift the slices of swordfish one by one, draining the marinade a little, and place them in an ovenproof dish. Bake at 180 degrees for no more than 5 minutes, so that the the fish releases the absorbed marinade. Stir in the swordfish carpaccio with green and pink pepper before serving.

15) Cod fillet with ginger

Ingredients:
- **Cod fillet 400 g**
- **Salt up to taste**
- **Black pepper to taste**
- **Extra virgin olive oil 50 g**
- **Lime zest 1**
- **Lime juice 10 g**
- **Fresh ginger (pulp) 20 g**
- **Mint a few leaves**

FOR THE RICE
- **Basmati rice 200 g**
- **Coconut milk 400 g**
- **Water 200 g**
- **Coarse salt 1 tbsp**
- **Cinnamon sticks 1**
- **Curry 1 tsp**

Grate the lime zest in a bowl and squeeze it into juice and pour 10 g into the same bowl. Peel the ginger and grate it, then collect the pulp with a spoon and place it in the bowl with the lime, pour in the olive oil and stir to mix the sauce. Take the cod fillets and place them on a baking sheet lined with parchment paper, salt them and spread the sauce on the surface. Bake in a preheated static oven at 220 ° for 25 minutes. Meanwhile, prepare the rice: pour the basmati rice into a pan, add the coconut milk, the coarse salt, the curry and a stick of cinnamon. Pour in the water, cover with the lid and bring to a boil, then lower the heat and cook for 15 minutes until the liquids are completely absorbed. When the rice has absorbed the liquids, turn off the heat and remove the cinnamon stick. Meanwhile, the cod will be cooked, take it out of the oven and serve it accompanied with the spiced basmati rice, garnishing with mint leaves.

Chapter 8: Dessert

1)   Buckwheat and dark chocolate cake

Ingredients:
- **100 g dates**
- **200 g buckwheat**
- **60 g bitter cocoa**
- **90 g 95% dark chocolate**
- **Grated orange peel to taste**
- **140 g tofu**
- **½ teaspoon of agar agar**

Soak the buckwheat for 24 hours, then drain and place in a sprouter. Rinse twice a day for 2-3 days, and as soon as it begins to sprout, place in the dryer basket at 42 ° for 8 hours. Blend the sprouted and dried buckwheat, dates, vanilla, and grated orange zest at maximum power. Add the tofu and continue blending. Separately, dissolve the agar agar in cold water and add to the mixture, mixing again. Add the dark chocolate in pieces and bring to a boil for a few minutes. Pour the mixture into a square shape, a level well, and store in the freezer for 3 hours. When the cake is ready, sprinkle with cocoa. Let it rest out of the freezer for at least half an hour.

2)   Apple and pear chutney with ginger and spices

Ingredients:
- 200 g of apples
- 200 g of golden onions
- 150 g of ripe but firm pears
- 40 g of whole cane sugar
- the juice of ½ lemon
- 140 ml of apple cider vinegar
- 4 cm of freshly chopped ginger
- ½ c of dried ginger powder
- ½ c of powdered cumin
- 100 ml of water, salt

Peel and cut the apples and pears into small pieces. Gather them in a thick-bottomed saucepan with the peeled and thinly sliced onions; add the rest of the ingredients and mix. Cook over medium heat for about 40 minutes, stirring often. If necessary, wet with a little water. Continue cooking until you have reached the consistency of a jam. Pour the still warm chutney into the jars and consume it within a week, keeping it in the refrigerator anyway.

3)   Rice cream flavored with ginger, turmeric and cinnamon

Ingredients:
- **250 g of gluten free rice biscuits**
- **80 g toasted hazelnuts**
- **500 g rice milk**
- **40 g starch**
- **3 cm cinnamon**
- **8 g of fresh turmeric**
- **20 g fresh ginger**
- **70 g brown sugar**
- **500 g of clean pumpkin**
- **100 g of cane sugar**
- **3 cm cinnamon**
- **water q.s.**

Chop the biscuits and half of the hazelnuts. Heat the rice milk with the cinnamon, which you will then remove. Grate the turmeric and ginger, put them in a kitchen towel, and squeeze them in the milk. When the milk is hot, add the starch and sugar, stirring with a whisk, and cook until the cream has thickened. Let it cool down. Dice the pumpkin and put it in a saucepan with the sugar, cinnamon, and 33 cl of water. Cook until the pumpkin is soft, then blend it with the blender and let it cool. Compose the cake in layers, alternating the biscuits, compote, and cream. As a topping, use the remaining chopped hazelnuts.

4) Beetroot brownies

Ingredients:
- **2 boiled beets**
- **200 g semi-wholemeal flour**
- **100 g dark chocolate (80-90%)**
- **50 g extra virgin olive oil**
- **50 g rice malt**
- **16 g yeast**
- **flaked almonds to taste**
- **1 handful of toasted hazelnuts**

Grate the beets, melt the chocolate in a bain-marie, add the oil, the malt, add the beets and mix everything. Add the sifted flour and baking powder. Mix well until the mixture is quite thick and soft. At this point, add the toasted hazelnuts and coarsely cut them with a knife. Transfer the dough to a previously greased square baking dish (about 30-40 cm). Bake in a preheated oven at 180 ° for about 30 minutes.

5)   Greedy glasses

Ingredients:
- **200 g of fresh blueberries**
- **4 heaping tablespoons of sugar-free blueberry jam**
- **2 tablespoons of organic apple juice**
- **500 ml of organic soy yogurt**
- **75 g of oat flakes**
- **75 g of pine nuts**

Clean and wash the blueberries. Blend them with half the yogurt and distribute them in 4 tall glasses. Heat the jam with the apple juice over low heat and divide it into glasses. Cover with the remaining yogurt and let it cool in the fridge for about an hour. Meanwhile, spread the oats and pine nuts on a baking sheet lined with parchment paper and toast them in the oven at 160 ° for about ten minutes, turning them now and then. Let them cool. Sprinkle with the mixture of pine nuts and oats, and serve immediately.

6) Soft blueberry pie

Ingredients:
- **250 g semi-wholemeal flour**
- **200 g of soy drink**
- **Juice and grated zest of 1 lemon**
- **16 g yeast**
- **50 g extra virgin olive oil**
- **50 g rice malt**
- **1 pinch of salt**
- **250 g blueberries**

Gather the flour, yeast, salt, lemon zest in a bowl; mix everything. Combine the soy drink, lemon juice, oil, and malt. Stir well until you get a velvety, lump-free consistency. Now add the blueberries. Transfer the dough to a previously greased loaf pan (about 30 cm). Bake in a preheated oven at 180 ° for about 30-40 minutes. The toothpick test is recommended to verify internal cooking. Let the cake cool before enjoying it. Keep inside a container for three days.

7) Lactose-free strawberry ice cream

Ingredients:
- **500 g of clean organic strawberries**
- **the juice of 1/2 lemon**
- **100 g of rice syrup**
- **260 ml of unsweetened rice milk**

Cut the strawberries, sprinkle them with the lemon juice and rice syrup, mix and let them rest in the refrigerator for half an hour. After this time, blend the mixture briefly with the rice milk. Leave it to cool for another half hour. Operate the ice cream maker and pour the mixture. It will take between 20 and 25 minutes to get good ice cream, be divided into cups or glasses, and be enjoyed immediately.

8) Pudding with pears and chocolate

Ingredients:
- **500 g vegetable soy drink**
- **3 large pears**
- **3 tablespoons of corn starch**
- **5 g of agar agar**
- **1 pinch of salt**
- **1 teaspoon of vanilla**
- **100 g 99% dark chocolate**
- **Chopped pistachio to taste**

Peel and wash the pears, cut them into slices, and steam them. Put the vegetable drink, agar agar, salt, vanilla, and the starch in a saucepan. Blend everything, add the cooked pears and blend again. Put on the fire, add the chopped chocolate and continue stirring. As soon as it starts to boil, turn off the heat. Put the chopped pistachios on the bottom of a pudding mold. Pour the mixture and let it cool for a few hours at room temperature. Then keep in the refrigerator.

9) Coconut balls

Ingredients:
- **1 cup of cashews**
- **5 dates**
- **grated coconut to taste**
- **rice milk to taste**

Pitted the dates, cut them into small pieces, put them in a robot together with the cashews, and blended them finely. With your hands, form balls, compacting them well. Let them rest for half an hour in the fridge. Meanwhile, mix a little coconut with two tablespoons of rice milk. Take the balls back and roll them in this mixture until they are evenly covered. Finally, put them in the paper cups and serve them.

10) Pear and cinnamon cake

Ingredients:
- 140 g of type 0 wheat flour
- 160 g of millet flour
- 1 p of sea salt
- ½ teaspoon of yeast
- 4 medium pears (2 quite ripe, 2 firmer)
- about 160 ml of rice milk
- 100 ml of oil
- 180 g of rice malt
- ½ teaspoon of ground cinnamon

Begin to heat the oven to 180 ° C. In the meantime, combine the wheat and millet flour in a bowl, the sea salt, yeast and mix well. Clean and peel the pears and cut only the two firmest into thin slices. Set the other two pears aside. Line a pan 20-22 cm in diameter with baking paper and arrange the pear slices on the bottom, overlapping them so that there are no gaps. Then cut the two more ripe pears into small pieces and place them in a mixer bowl. Add the rice milk, the oil, the malt, and the cinnamon and blend well until you obtain a smooth mixture which you will combine with the dry ingredients previously mixed, mixing briefly. Pour everything into the pan on the slices of pear. Bake and cook for 40-45 minutes. Finally, remove the cake from the oven, let it cool for 5-10 minutes before serving it with a vegetable cream sauce sweetened with a few tablespoons of rice malt of about.

11) Vegan apple pie

Ingredients:
- **3 apples**
- **250 g of type 1 wheat flour**
- **60 g of raisins**
- **60 g of almonds**
- **About 250 ml of apple juice**
- **50 g of corn oil**
- **1 teaspoon of cinnamon**
- **grated lemon peel**
- **1/2 sachet of baking powder**
- **1 pinch of salt**

Soak the raisins. In a bowl, put the dry ingredients: flour, chopped almonds, lemon peel, cinnamon, and salt; stir with care. In another, gather the apple juice, the oil, the raisins, the peeled and chopped apples; mix them well, and mix them with the other container's contents. Mix the mixture carefully, roll it out in a pan; bake at 180 degrees for about 50-60 minutes. Check the cooking with a toothpick: if it comes out dry, turn off the oven. Let the cake rest briefly, unmold it, and let it cool completely on a wire rack before enjoying.

12) Plum and fig balls

Ingredients:
- **100 g of pitted dried plums**
- **100 g of dried figs**
- **50 g of chopped hazelnuts**
- **cocoa**

Put the plums, figs, and hazelnuts in the mixer. Knead them until you get a homogeneous mixture from which you will obtain slightly larger balls of hazelnuts with the shell. Roll them well in cocoa and immediately arrange them in paper cups. They are ready to be served!

13) Cookies with apple heart

Ingredients:

For the shortcrust pastry
- **an egg**
- **100 g of cane sugar**
- **half a bag of yeast**
- **semi-wholemeal flour to taste**
- **a coffee glass of extra virgin olive oil**
- **grated orange peel**

For the apple filling
- **3 apples**
- **2 teaspoons of powdered ginger**
- **the juice of half a lemon**
- **2 tablespoons of brown sugar**

In a bowl, put the egg, brown sugar, grated orange peel, and olive oil. Mix the ingredients with a fork in a circular and continuous pattern until you get a homogeneous and creamy mixture. Stir in the yeast and mix.

At this point, add the sifted flour a little at a time, always mixing it with a fork in the bowl. You will see the dough gradually transform, acquire body and shape while remaining soft. For the recipe's success, this is an important step: consider mixing the flour at the rate of a spoon at a time until your liquid and creamy dough become more compact but not hard. Transfer it to a lightly floured pastry board and knead. When it no longer sticks to your hands, your pastry will be ready. Give it a ball shape and place it in the refrigerator for 30 minutes.

Peel and dice the apples, put them in a bowl, add the lemon juice, the ginger powder, and the sugar. Mix well and pour into a non-stick pan. Cook for about 10 minutes (the time varies depending on the quality of the apples chosen) over moderate heat until you get a fragrant and creamy mixture. Leave to cool. Take the pastry, roll it out finely and form circles you will use to shape your cookies. Everything is ready to assemble the ingredients: you will need a bowl with a little water to seal the edges of the biscuits and prevent the contents from escaping: take a pastry base, put the apple filling in the center, with your index finger wet with water moisten the edges of the two pastry bases; then seal the two edges by pressing on them to push the filling towards the center and prevent it from coming out during cooking. With the help of a fork, decorate the edge with light pressure. Repeat until all ingredients are used up. Put the biscuits in a baking tray covered with parchment paper and bake them for 15 minutes at 180 °. A sprinkle of powdered sugar and they are ready ... soft, healthy, and very tasty.

14) Carrot cake

Ingredients:
- **200 g of wholemeal flour**
- **80 g of almonds**
- **80 g of raisins**
- **200 g of carrots**
- **100 g of rice malt**
- **4 tablespoons of sunflower oil**
- **1 orange**
- **3 tablespoons of corn starch**
- **1 teaspoon of yeast**
- **½ teaspoon of natural vanilla**
- **soya milk**
- **1 pinch of salt**

Wash the orange, grate the zest and squeeze the juice. Put the first in a bowl together with the flour, finely ground almonds, starch, yeast, vanilla, and salt. Stir. Mix the oil, malt, and orange juice in a bowl. Gradually add them to the dry ingredients. Complete with grated carrots and rinsed raisins. If the dough is too firm, dilute it with a little soy milk. Line a square mold of about 20 cm on each side with baking paper. Transfer the mixture, level it, and bake at 180 degrees for about 45 minutes. Check the cooking with a toothpick, which must come out dry. Let the cake cool in the pan, turn it out of the mold, and let it cool.

15) Chocolate cake

Ingredients:
- **80 grams of unsweetened cocoa powder**
- **100 grams of coconut flour**
- **300 g 0 flour**
- **100 gr of hazelnuts**
- **150 ml of seed oil**
- **350 grams of rice or soy milk**
- **150 g of cane sugar**
- **a sachet of vanilla yeast for cakes**

In a blender, finely chop the hazelnuts and place them in a large bowl. Add the unsweetened cocoa, coconut flour and flour, sugar, and vanilla yeast. Mix these ingredients vigorously with your hands, mixing them well together. Then add the vegetable milk and mix the mixture with the help of a spoon. Also, add the seed oil: the result must be a soft, not liquid compound. Line a cake pan with parchment paper and spread the cocoa mixture starting from the center towards the outer sides, and spread all the product well in the pan. You can put some chopped hazelnuts or almonds on top of the cake for decoration. Place in a preheated oven at 180 ° for 40 minutes. Remove from the oven and sprinkle the cake while still hot with a coconut flour cascade or, if you prefer, powdered sugar. Few genuine ingredients that, when mixed, give a great result. Excellent for those intolerant to dairy products and to let everyone discover a lively and tasty vegan diet.

Chapter 9: Sauces, toppings and condiments

1) Black Cabbage Pesto

Ingredients:
- **350 g of black cabbage**
- **50 g of walnut kernels**
- **1 heaping tablespoon of pine nuts**
- **1 clove of garlic**
- **5 tablespoons of oil**
- **a pinch of salt**

Clean and steam the cabbage for 5-6 minutes. Blend it with the walnuts, garlic, pine nuts, oil, and salt, helping you if needed with a little water kept aside. It was excellent for dressing pasta, cereals, rice, and polenta, filling for crepes, sandwiches, and savory scones, or simply spreading on croutons for an unusual and tasty appetizer.

Variant
You can replace the black cabbage with savoy cabbage and add a handful of almonds instead of walnuts and pine nuts.

2) Dried fig and orange jam

Ingredients:
- **150 g of dried figs**
- **5 oranges**
- **200 g of whole cane sugar**

Wash the figs and soak them for about an hour. In the meantime, peel an orange, remove the zest of almost all the white part and cut it into strips. Then dip it in a saucepan with a little boiling water for 1 minute, change the water, and repeat for a second time: this procedure will help you remove the peel's bitter taste. Peel the other oranges cut them all into cubes, remove the seeds, and pour the pulp into a pot with the peel and brown sugar. Bring to a boil and cook for about 10 minutes. Add the figs cut small and thin, and cook until the mixture becomes thick. Pour the jam into the sterilized jars and proceed with the preferred storage method. Once cold, keep the jars in a cool and dry place and use the contents after a month.

3)   Dried fruit chocolates

Ingredients:
- **200 g dark chocolate (99%)**
- **3 tablespoons of goji berries**
- **3 tablespoons of sliced almonds**
- **3 tablespoons of walnuts**
- **6 dried figs**

Soak the goji berries in water for about 10 minutes; when they are soft, drain. Cut the figs into slices. Separately, melt the chocolate. At this point, take a spoonful of chocolate and create some discs on the parchment paper, then place the dried fruit on the chocolate and wait for everything to cool. Store in the refrigerator.

4)   Fragrant pumpkin jam

Ingredients:
- **1 kg of pumpkin**
- **150 g of whole cane sugar**
- **the grated peel and the juice of 1 lemon**
- **1 teaspoon of cinnamon**

Remove the seeds but not the skin from the pumpkin and cut them into small pieces. Let it soften for 5 minutes in a steamer: you will also use the resulting water. With its cooking water, put it in a thick-bottomed pot together with all the ingredients, taking care to set aside half of the grated lemon zest, and cook over low heat, stirring often. After about 30-40 minutes, the pumpkin will have completely undone, and the skin will tend to disappear for the most part; whatever remains will give your preserves a special crunchy touch. Just before potting, add the remaining lemon peel to keep all its scent intact. Evaluate the consistency of the jam and put the jam in sterilized jars.

5)   Eggplant and ginger jam

Ingredients:
- **1 kg of eggplant**
- **100 g of whole cane sugar**
- **50 g of fresh grated ginger**
- **the juice of 1 lemon**
- **1 chopped red pepper**
- **1 cup of water**

Cut the eggplant into cubes. Put 1 cup of water in a saucepan and bring it to a boil. Add the eggplant, ginger, and chili. Cook over low heat for about 30 minutes, stirring constantly. Add the lemon juice and sugar, continuing to mix for another 15 minutes. Blend the mixture with an immersion blender or a puree and pour it still boiling into the previously sterilized jars, close and proceed with sterilization.

6)   Homemade ketchup

Ingredients:
- 2 cups of cherry tomatoes
- 5-6 dried tomatoes
- 1 teaspoon of brown sugar
- 1 teaspoon of lemon juice
- 2 teaspoons of apple or rice cider vinegar
- Himalayan salt
- Tabasco

Pour the dried tomatoes in hot water and half the vinegar for 15 minutes. Wash the fresh ones and dry them. Halve them and put them in the mixer with the soaked ones, which you will have squeezed and chopped. Blend until creamy. Add the sugar, lemon juice, tabasco, salt, and the rest of the vinegar. Mix carefully. Transfer the mixture to a jar and keep it in the fridge for a few days.

7)   Catalan cream

Ingredients:
- 500 ml of soy milk
- 90 g of brown sugar + another 4 tablespoons
- 4 yolks
- 30 g of corn starch
- 1 piece of cinnamon
- ½ untreated lemon zest

Heat the milk with the cinnamon and lemon zest in a saucepan. Meanwhile, beat the egg yolks in a bowl with 90 g of cane sugar and corn starch. Before the milk boils, remove it from the heat and filter it, removing the cinnamon and lemon zest. Pour the liquid over the beaten egg yolks. Mix well with a whisk and transfer the mixture to the saucepan. Put it back on the stove and heat it over low heat, always stirring with a whisk. Allow about 2 more minutes of cooking from boiling. Remove the cream from the heat and distribute it in individual cups. Sprinkle with the remaining sugar, caramelize with the special tool, or briefly pass the bowls under the oven grill.

8)   Orange pesto

Ingredients:
- **2 oranges**
- **100 g of almonds**
- **50 g of capers**
- **a bunch of parsley**
- **a few leaves of fresh marjoram**
- **a bunch of oregano**
- **the grated rind of an orange and a lemon**
- **Salt to taste.**
- **extra virgin olive oil as needed**

Grate the peel of one of the two oranges and set it aside together with the grated peel of a lemon. Eliminate the white part from the oranges taking care to keep only the pulp, also eliminating the internal seeds. Put the pulp collected in the immersion blender's container and add the almonds, parsley, a pinch of oregano, and a few marjoram leaves. Adjust with a drizzle of oil and a little salt. Blend all the ingredients until you get a homogeneous and compact pulp. Season with salt if necessary. A fresh and very fragrant pesto; use it to dress pasta and cereals, salads, or croutons.

9) Spiced pumpkin jam

Ingredients:
- **1 kg of pumpkin**
- **3 tablespoons of 100% malt rice**
- **1 cup of almonds**
- **2 teaspoons of vanilla powder**
- **2 teaspoons of cinnamon**
- **4 cardamom capsules**
- **the juice and zest of 1 grated lemon**
- **2 teaspoons of agar-agar**

Clean the pumpkin, cut it into small pieces and make a puree that you will cook for 15 minutes with the juice and peel of the lemon and the cardamom seeds deprived of the shell. Continue cooking for another 20-30 minutes, mixing often and skimming if necessary. Add the chopped almonds, malt, cinnamon, and vanilla powder to the mixture. Mix well and add the agar-agar that you have previously dissolved in a little water and left to rest for at least 15 minutes. Continue to cook over high heat, stirring well for another 5 minutes, then put the jam in sterilized jars.

10) Lemon-scented apple jam

Ingredients:
- **1 kg of apples**
- **2 lemons**
- **2 tablespoons of 100% malt rice**
- **1 teaspoon of cinnamon**

Wash apples and lemons and dry them. Cut the apples into quarters without peeling them but removing only the core and seeds, then slice them very thinly. Cut the lemons with the peel into small pieces and remove all the seeds. Put the apples and lemons in a pot with the water and cook for 15 minutes over high heat. Lower the heat and continue cooking until the apple and lemons are crushed, forming a thick mixture. Use a puree or a mixer to blend the jam, then add the malt and cinnamon. Finally, raise the heat and finish cooking over high heat and stirring for a few minutes. Try the saucer test and keep. You can also decide to cook the lemons without the peel, adding the desired percentage of peel to the mixture just before potting.

11) Curry tofu cream

Ingredients:
- **300 g of tofu**
- **1 onion**
- **1 apple**
- **1 teaspoon of spicy curry**
- **2 teaspoons of sweet curry**
- **vegetable broth**
- **3 tablespoons of oil**
- **salt**

Finely chop the onion and put it in a pan covered with broth. Cook it over low heat, with the lid on, until it is soft. If necessary, gradually add more hot broth. Meanwhile, put the tofu in a saucepan, cover it with water and let it boil slowly. Turn off the heat and let it cool. Wash the apple and core it, cut it into wedges and add it to the onion. Mix the two types of curry in a little broth and pour them into the pan. Stir well and cook for another 5 minutes. Turn off the heat and let it rest. Combine the diced tofu and the curry sauce in a blender. Add the oil and a little salt. Blend them until smooth, helping you if needed with a little broth. When the sauce is creamy, serve it spread on bread, or use it to season cooked cereals or vegetables.

12) Yogurt mayonnaise

Ingredients:
- **200 g of soy yogurt**
- **oil, lemon juice**
- **1 pinch of mustard powder**
- **salt**

Put the yogurt in a container with high sides. It will gradually pour in the oil (one tablespoon at a time, it will take four to five) and whip the sauce with the hand blender. When the mayonnaise is thick, add a few drops of lemon juice, mustard, and salt. Leave it in the fridge for a couple of hours before enjoying it with a vegetable salad or roasted vegetables.

13) Aubergine sauce

Ingredients:
•2 medium-sized eggplants
•1 clove of garlic
•abundant basil
•1 sprig of parsley
•a pinch of grated lemon zest
•20 g of pine nuts
•extra virgin olive oil
•whole sea salt

In a saucepan, bring lightly salted water to a boil. In the meantime, clean, peel and divide the aubergine pulp into chunks. Blanch the aubergines for 3 minutes, then blend them until they are reduced to a smooth and homogeneous cream. Season with salt and season with oil and a small piece of lemon zest. With a mixer's help, prepare an emulsified sauce based on garlic, basil, a few parsley leaves, extra virgin olive oil, and salt. Serve the aubergine sauce with the basil emulsion and the pine nuts toasted in a pan on top.

14) Maple syrup sauce

Ingredients:
- **250 g of maple syrup**
- **50 ml of vegetable cream**
- **1 pinch of sea salt**
- **2 tablespoons of brown sugar**
- **1 teaspoon of natural vanilla extract**
- **1 tablespoon of corn starch**

Gather the maple syrup, vegetable cream, salt, brown sugar, and vanilla extract in a small thick-bottomed saucepan. Stir and bring to a boil. Lower the heat and cook for 10-15 minutes, stirring often. Add the starch, dissolved in 2 tablespoons of water, and continue cooking for a few more minutes until the sauce has thickened. Remove from heat and set aside to cool.

15) Ginger and avocado sauce

Ingredients:
2 ripe avocados
the juice of 1 lemon
1 clove of garlic
2 tablespoons of chopped walnuts
1 tablespoon of fresh grated ginger
1 pinch of salt
125 grams of soy yogurt

Peel the avocados and pit them. Mash the pulp with a fork and sprinkle it immediately with the filtered lemon juice to prevent it from blackening. Add the crushed garlic and grated ginger. Finally, gently stir in the yogurt and add salt. To speed up the timing, you can put everything in the mixer.

Conclusion

It is undoubtedly the most precious and impressive exchange surface between organism and environment. It regulates the absorption of nutrients, which is essential to guarantee our survival and modulates a very numerous series of functions, generally microscopic, which allow us to remain healthy and why not also happy. We are talking about the intestine, an organ for a long time, only considered a "tube attached to the stomach, " which has been in the last two decades. However, it proved to be a key element in maintaining the balance of organic functions. Therefore, it will be simplistic to imagine him engaged "only" in the absorption of precious nutrients and the elimination of waste substances. Still, it will be necessary to consider him involved in regulating immune function, in the management of numerous metabolic functions, and the maintenance of physical and mental well-being. A healthy intestine is therefore essential in maintaining a healthy body. And to take care of it, you need to start right from the choices at the table.

www.ingramcontent.com/pod-product-compliance
Lightning Source LLC
Chambersburg PA
CBHW061324120726
48001CB00002B/686